Foundations for Operating Department Practice

Practice
2nd edition

Foundations for Operating Department Practice

Essential theory for practice

2nd edition

Edited by Hannah Abbott and Helen Booth

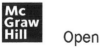
Open University Press

Open University Press
McGraw Hill
Unit 4,
Foundation Park
Roxborough Way
Maidenhead
SL6 3UD

email: emea_uk_ireland@mheducation.com
world wide web: www.mheducation.co.uk

First edition published 2014
First published in this second edition 2024

A catalogue record of this book is available from the British Library

ISBN-13: 9780335251025
ISBN-10: 0335251021
eISBN: 9780335251032

Typeset by Transforma Pvt. Ltd., Chennai, India

Praise page

"I would list this as 'highly recommended' to all Student ODPs. A book written by ODPs for ODPs.

It's vital to support practice-based learning with the underpinning requirements of an all-degree profession. This edition links very well to the current BSc Curriculum in Operating Department Practice and the updated Health and Care Professions Standards of Proficiency for ODPs. Within this book, students will gain great support with the challenges of learning within the Higher Education Environment. The non-clinical knowledge, skills, and expectations of the modern ODP are excellently covered in several chapters.

It is my belief that this book should be included on the reading list of all ODP programmes and Perioperative HEI Programmes."

John Dade RODP, PGCMedEd, Immediate Past President –
The Association for Perioperative Practice

"This text offers an eclectic mix of topics which reflects the breath of operating department practice. Each author provides context specific to Operating Department Practitioners (ODPs), whilst exploring relevant theories and contemporary material. In some cases, authors draw upon seminal texts and their application to perioperative care and operating department practice. With a range of relevant sources and further reading, alongside 'stop and think' moments which enrich the reading experience, this book is suitable for both pre-registration learners and post registration practitioners to explore theory and concepts which are related directly to the role of the ODP and the broader scope of professional practice in contemporary healthcare."

Helen Lowes, National AHP Education and Training Lead
for Operating Department Practitioners, NHS England, UK

"I really like this updated edition. The experience of the authors - all operating department practitioners - comes through in the text. Each chapter is clearly written in a way that merges the broadness of theory that ODPs need to know and the demands of the clinical practice in one of the most complicated departments in the modern hospital. Unlike other books, the authors achieve this balance by offering theory to support an understanding of practice and sharing their practice experiences to contextualise the theory. This book is also different to others, as it celebrates

Contents

List of contributors

Hannah Abbott (Editor) MSc, PG Cert, PGCE, BSc (Hons), ODP, MCODP, FCODP
Head of College, College of Health and Care Professions, Birmingham City University

Helen Booth (Editor) MA (Bioethics), BSc (Hons), Cert Ed, ODP, FCODP
College of Operating Department Practice

Rebecca Daly BSc (Hons), DipHE ODP, PGCAP, SFHEA
Lecturer in Operating Department Practice, University of Hull

Michael Donnellon MBA, MA (Ed), PG Cert, FHEA, ODP, MCODP, FCODP
Former Senior Lecturer in Operating Department Practice, University of Central Lancashire, College of Operating Department Practice

Laura Garbett MSc Profprac (Healthcare), LLB(Hons), PGCLTHE, DipHE ODP, FHEA, SEDA
Senior Lecturer Operating Department Practice, Birmingham City University

Andrew Gulley BSc (Hons), FHEA, ODP, MCODP, PGCE Learning Technologies and Cert Ed.
Deputy Head of Operating Department Practice, University of Leicester

Penny Joyce EdD, MEd, BA Ed, PFHEA, ODP
Former Principal Lecturer, University of Portsmouth
Former Independent Member, Education and Training Committee, Health and Care Professions Council

William Kilvington D. Univ., ODP, FCODP, FRCA
Patient Safety Lead, College of Operating Department Practitioners

Christine Mahoney BSc (Hons), PGCE, ODP
Former Senior Lecturer and Course Director (Perioperative Programmes), Faculty of Health and Social Care, London South Bank University

Susan Parker EdD, MA(Ed), PG Dip, BSc (Open), ODP, MCODP
Senior Operating Department Practitioner, Practice Development Team, PACU, University Hospitals North Midlands

Daniel Rodger MA (Ethics), BSc (Hons), PGCLTHE, ODP
Senior Lecturer, Operating Department Practice, Institute of Health and Social Care, London South Bank University

Keith Underwood ODP, FCODP, DipICM
Former Medical Devices Safety Officer (MDSO)

Stephen Wordsworth EdD, MSc, PG Cert, BA (Hons), Cert Ed, ODP, MCODP, FCODP
Deputy Dean, College of Health, Psychology and Social Care, University of Derby

Foreword

I am delighted to write the foreword for this book, as the Operating Department Practitioner (ODP) profession continues to grow in strength, with an emphasis on improved patient care, and has a positive, professional reputation.

Following a public consultation, July 2021 saw the Health and Care Professions Council (HCPC) decide to increase the threshold level at which students would qualify to be able to register as ODPs to that of having been awarded a degree. The consultation process showed support for this decision, and it was seen as aligning with the HCPC's goals to improve the safety of patients and service users and advance the ODP role as a profession. From 2024, the move to an all-graduate profession will see the HCPC approve only those ODP education programmes that lead to a degree. We know that the evidence shows, across the health professions, that being educated to degree level ensures that members of staff are well equipped to provide high-quality, safe care. This also prepares them to take the lead, inform and develop the delivery of health services, both in the perioperative environment and beyond, and be involved in decision-making and policy development across multiprofessional teams.

In the inspirational foreword to the first edition of this book, Bill Kilvington set out the history of the profession from its beginnings, which, if we look at the key role ODPs are playing in perioperative and other environments in the NHS today, is almost unrecognizable. We still see and hear about staffing shortages, as highlighted by the Bevan report in 1989, but we have also seen how ODPs have modernized and stepped up in other critical care arenas during the COVID-19 pandemic, for example. No longer a profession hidden behind the closed doors of operating theatres, ODPs have developed their practice into a range of settings, such as intensive care units, high dependency departments and emergency departments.

ODPs are recognized as vital members of multidisciplinary teams. The profession has been regulated by the HCPC since 2004 and, in 2017 (in England), joined the 13 other professions known as Allied Health Professionals. This has led to wider recognition and, more recently, a public consultation to consider the potential for ODPs to be able to supply and administer medicines using patient group directions (PGDs). Currently, ODPs can supply and administer medicines using patient-specific directions (PSDs). While these are useful in many clinical settings and will often be sufficient to meet the needs of patients and service users, they also have intrinsic limitations. If it is decided that ODPs should be able to administer medicines under a PGD, this has the potential to improve both the timely manner of drug administration and patient outcomes. ODPs will be able to further complement the work of multiprofessional teams and improve the treatment of patients and their experience.

It is the evolution of the role in ways such as this that have brought about the career progression from its start to the point where now several roles have opened up in the perioperative environment, such as in education, leadership or management and as anaesthesia associates. The roles outside this environment are also varied and include those of surgical care practitioner (a hybrid role, working as part of the medical surgical team in outpatient departments, wards and operating theatre) and advanced clinical practitioner.

I'd like to finish with an extract from the 'NHS Constitution for England' (Department of Health and Social Care 2023) to remind us of the role ODPs play in the NHS to ensure the realization of its vital, primary value, which is that healthcare is:

> available to all irrespective of gender, race, disability, age, sexual orientation, religion, belief, gender reassignment, pregnancy and maternity or marital or civil partnership status. The service is designed to improve, prevent, diagnose and treat both physical and mental health problems with equal regard. It has a duty to each and every individual that it serves and must respect their human rights.

Deborah Robinson MSc, Dip HE ODP, ODP
Interim Dean of the Faculty of Health Science
University of Hull

Department of Health and Social Care (DHSC) (2021) The NHS Constitution for England. London: DHSC.

Preface

This book has been written to support pre- and post-registration Operating Department Practitioners (ODPs), both during their undergraduate studies and throughout their professional careers. It has been written by ODPs from academic and clinical settings throughout the UK and, while the content may also be relevant to other professionals, it is designed to meet the specific needs of ODPs.

As you will have read in the Foreword, the role of ODP has undergone rapid development over the past 30 years. It is important to note that for it to have become established as an independent profession with a unique body of knowledge in this short time is a remarkable achievement. While our clinical knowledge and skills have developed, this is not the most significant marker of the development of the profession; rather, it is the professional qualities, attributes, commitment to evidence-based care and an understanding of the wider context of care that qualifies us as registered practitioners in our own right. In recognition of these developments and to support the transition to an all-graduate profession, it was timely to write a book that encapsulates the skills and attributes in the unique context of the ODP profession.

This text does not include instruction in clinical skills, as there are existing texts that address these and, in fact, the dynamic nature of the environment means that journal articles are the best sources of information to keep your clinical skills up to date, as they reflect the current evidence. The focus of this text, therefore, is on the fundamental professional knowledge and skills that enable ODPs to deliver effective, compassionate and evidence-based care to patients, and the continual development of this professional knowledge and skills. Each chapter explores the underpinning principles of a topic area, then links these to practice, with a clear focus on the application of knowledge through practice-based examples and 'Stop and think' boxes to help you relate the principles to your own practice. This text provides you with information, but we also hope that it will act as a catalyst, encouraging you to question practices and undertake further reading about the subject areas included here.

While this book includes a number of distinctly different topics, you will find that links can be made between them. You will also find that the authors have written their chapters in slightly different styles. As editors we have welcomed this as we feel it is important that each chapter uses the language most suited to the given topic, plus we wanted to show that there are different approaches to written work to encourage you to develop your own style of academic and professional writing.

In this book, we have sought to provide you with a good overview of the fundamental topics. However, they are extensive, so undertaking wider reading is important to develop your knowledge of them further and to update it as new information is discovered. You will find that each chapter is supported by evidence and there is a references and further reading section at the end of each one that will serve as a good starting point for your wider reading. The evidence supporting the chapters in this book is drawn from both contemporary and classical sources, so you can understand the contexts in which the knowledge was developed.

We hope that you will enjoy this book and find it helpful as you develop your career in this exciting and dynamic profession.

1 Developing your learning as an Operating Department Practitioner

Andrew Gulley

Key topics

- Exploring learning styles and theories
- Blended, remote and distance learning approaches
- How to use learning outcomes to enhance your learning
- Assessment and revision strategies
- Tools to support learning, including portfolios

Introduction

The aim of this chapter is to take you through a back-to-basics perspective on the teaching, learning and assessment approaches used in higher education (HE) for both new learners and those practitioners returning to learning. The skills, practices and attitudes fundamental to operating department practice are learned from the achievement, integration and critical application of knowledge and understanding, cognitive/intellectual skills, key/transferable skills and practical skills gained from the whole educational experience (College of Operating Department Practitioners (CODP) 2018).

By exploring the key topics in this chapter, you will be able to develop effective learning plans, strategies and behaviours to meet professional standards and, ultimately, be successful in your studies. It is acknowledged that some content will already be known by experienced learners; however, the focus of the chapter is on giving support to all Operating Department Practitioner (ODP) learners in their ongoing professional education.

Why is this relevant?

Whether you are new to learning or returning to it, some adjustments need to be made to how you plan your time and to the new experience of life at university, which can be complex and confusing. There will be many opportunities to develop your skills and become a successful learner. Studying operating department practice also brings with it a unique learning experience – that of clinical practice.

This is sometimes viewed as the vocational aspect of the curriculum, with learners linking academic theory and knowledge to their application in practice. When undertaking your pre- or post-registration ODP studies, therefore, you will be learning in both university and practice settings.

To use the time you have for study as effectively as possible, it is important to understand the approaches taken to teaching, learning and assessment. Then, by learning to learn, you can engage with them in ways that will enhance both your personal development and your learning. By understanding these approaches, plus the skills, practices and attitudes fundamental to operating department practice, the whole educational experience will become pleasant, engaging and rewarding.

This chapter provides learners with an insight into and understanding of the key academic norms and values relating to teaching, learning and assessment, primarily in the HE setting, though the skills of learning are central to your ongoing development throughout your career as an ODP.

Learning styles

ODPs are individuals and so assimilate and process information in different ways. Equally, in a diverse group of learners, there will be a range of learning 'styles'. Most people recognize that learners will differ in this way and in their preferences for teaching techniques, finding some rather than others enable them to grasp the subject, whether in academic or clinical practice settings (D'Amore et al. 2011). While studying, therefore, you may learn the material in several different ways, such as by seeing and hearing, reflecting and acting on your learning, thinking logically and instinctively, and analysing and visualizing the information being presented. This should be done in a continual manner to ensure that development takes place in a progressive way, measured against your learning objectives. Having regular successes in the process of learning is important as this allows achievements to be recognized and builds confidence in your ability to succeed.

Learning styles group common characteristics in learning that help you to learn effectively. The different styles involve variations in the ways we represent experiences to ourselves internally, the ways we recall information, and even the words we choose, all of which have a bearing on assessment outcomes and achievements. Having an insight into learning styles can help you to develop appropriate strategies to improve your academic development and performance (Horton et al. 2012). However, if you were to conduct a literature search for the term 'learning styles' you would find more than 70 different variations on the fundamental models first proposed. This suggests that educators advocate their use, but there is no real evidence to support the use of learning styles. The role of educators is to deliver effective and coherent teaching and, hence, present subjects, skills or theories in a combination of different pedagogical approaches that enable students to achieve the best levels of retention of knowledge and experiential learning (Roher and Pashler 2012).

It is worth exploring the basic concepts of learning styles. For an insight into them, let us now look briefly at two common and fundamental examples, from which many other learning styles are derived. These are the VARK and Kolb's models.

The VARK and Kolb's learning styles models

The acquisition of knowledge through experience is associated with different learning styles, so here we consider the concepts of visual, auditory, reading/writing and kinaesthetic modes of learning, or, VARK (Cherry 2023) and those of Kolb (1984).

Cherry (2023) suggests that the VARK modalities reflect the lifelong learning experiences of learners. The VARK learning styles inventory not only tells you what your preferred style is but also offers specific strategies suited to you for teaching, learning, revision and assessment. In a classroom setting or in the operating theatre, for example, you will be using your senses to assimilate and process information in different ways. In a classroom setting, the tutor may present an image of an anatomical structure or talk about a patient care situation. In contrast, in the perioperative environment, you might look at and identify specific internal anatomy. Whatever the context or situation of the learning experience, therefore, you will be using sensory modalities – that is, visual (seeing the image), aural (listening to your practice educator (PE) or tutor), reading/writing (taking notes in a lecture) and kinaesthetic activities (hands-on care; Hydrie et al. 2021). The VARK modalities, characteristics and examples of learning strategies are shown in Table 1.1. It should be recognized, however, that research suggests most learners are multimodal in their approach to learning styles, so they cannot be pigeonholed into only one learning style.

Stop and think

Look at Table 1.1 and consider which of the techniques you have used for learning in the past. If you have not studied for a while, which option helps most you when you need to remember things? Consider how you can use this important information about your learning preferences to support your studies.

Table 1.1 The VARK modalities, characteristics and learning strategies

Modalities	Characteristics and learning strategies
Visual	This is a preference for information presented visually and using symbols to represent words. Strategies include the depiction of information in maps, spider diagrams, charts, graphs, flow charts, labelled diagrams, symbolic arrows, circles and using symbols.
Auditory	This is a preference for information that is heard or spoken. Learn best from lectures, group discussion, radio, email, using phone, speaking, webchat and talking things through.
Reading/writing	This preference emphasizes text-based input and output, so strategies include reading and writing in all its forms, but especially manuals, reports, essays and assignments.
Kinaesthetic	A preference related to being able to experience and practise to learn (whether simulated or real). The best strategy is to learn by doing.

Source: Adapted from Cherry (2023)

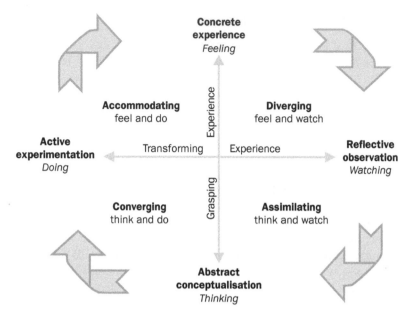

Figure 1.1 Kolb's learning styles model
Source: Adapted from Kurt (2022)

Kolb's learning styles (1984; Hydrie et al. 2021) model draws on the cognitive personality styles assessed by, for example, the classic Myers-Briggs Type Indicator, a psychological personality test that has been used for more than 50 years and been the subject of extensive validity and reliability studies (D'Amore et al. 2011).

To illustrate the theory, Kolb (1984) combined a horizontal axis of perceiving (transforming an experience) with a vertical axis of processing (grasping an experience). These axes create four quadrants, delineating distinct learning modes that represent different styles of learning (see Figure 1.1).

Divergers	learn by combining concrete experience with reflective observation to create a learning style that can view concrete situations from various viewpoints.
Assimilators	thrive by reflecting on abstract concepts and putting the information in logical form.
Convergers	take abstract ideas and actively experiment to find practical uses for the information by finding solutions to problems.
Accommodators	take concrete experiences mixed with active experimentation in a hands-on experience.

You will probably find that you engage with all Kolb's learning styles by, for example, using simulation in advanced trauma life support (accommodating), linking your lecture notes to practice (assimilating), engaging with problem-based learning scenarios in the classroom (converging) and observing and reflecting on clinical practice (diverging).

Kolb's model of experiential learning

As an ODP, a lot of your learning will be drawn from your educational and practice experiences. You can develop the learning gained from these experiences further if you identify where you are in terms of your learning cycle. Kolb's (1984) model presents experiential learning as a cyclical process, whereby knowledge is created through the transformation of experiences in the stages in the cycle. This model fits well with the profession's body of knowledge, identified in the pre-registration ODP curriculum, which advocates that cognitive/intellectual skills, key/transferable skills and practical skills are gained from the whole educational experience (HCPC 2017a; CODP 2018).

Kolb's theory provides a rationale for a variety of learning methods, including independent learning, learning by doing, work-based learning and problem-based learning. These methods are all necessary if learning is to be consolidated and implemented in practice.

Kolb describes the cycle of experiential learning as having four stages (see Figure 1.2). The idea is that, as you move through the cycle, you first have the immediate, concrete experience, which leads to reflection and observations on the experience. These reflections are then assimilated and linked with previous knowledge, to be translated into abstract concepts or theories, which result in a process of active experimentation, with new ways and actions tried out so that the experience can be tested and explored.

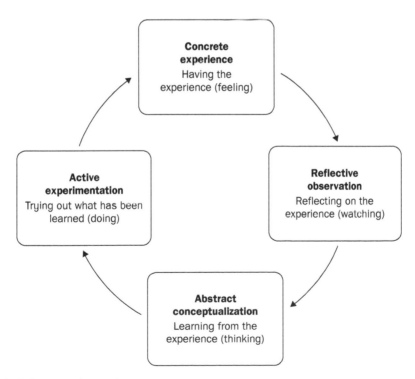

Figure 1.2 Kolb's learning cycle

Source: Adapted from Kolb (1984)

To give an example of how Kolb's learning cycle could be used in practice, consider an ODP who has cared for a very anxious patient undergoing general anaesthesia (concrete experience). Afterwards, the ODP reflects on what took place (reflective observation), then discusses events with their PE and other colleagues. The ODP then considers this in the context of their previous experiences, as well as published policies, good practice and the literature on this subject (abstract conceptualization). Based on these reflections and wider reading, the ODP then identifies some strategies and changes that they can apply to similar clinical situations in the future (active experimentation). After doing that, the ODP can assess the efficacy of these strategies by working through the cycle again.

Over the course of a programme of study, there will generally be a balance of teaching and learning methods, so all learners will have an opportunity to learn using their preferred learning style. Such a balance will mean that learners will also be exposed to approaches that they like less but these will have the benefit of providing them with other, new sets of learning strategies. Though they may not be comfortable with them initially, these methods and strategies may help them to be successful in their academic and vocational studies. Individual learners will still, of course, have their preferred learning styles and these will influence and guide their learning. If you have an insight into what your learning style is, this can help you to develop appropriate strategies to improve your academic development. The VARK and Kolb models provide a comprehensive analysis of learners' learning styles and suggest learning strategies appropriate to those styles, but the models should only be used as an aid, not as a prescriptive method of learning.

Stop and think

Thinking back to your own experiences, what type of learning sessions have you found most beneficial?

Look at Kolb's learning styles and characteristics and identify how your own preferences relate to the different styles that Kolb suggests.

Educational learning theories

The use of educational learning theories can inform teaching strategies and the selection of different learning resources. Ultimately, it is the learning activities in which learners engage that determine what they will learn.

There are four common educational learning theories that can be applied to ODP education.

Behaviourist theory

Behaviourist theory is primarily and historically associated with Pavlov's dogs, in 'classical conditioning', and Skinner's rats, in 'operant conditioning' (Sarafino 2008). Most of the evidence for this theory comes from experiments performed using animals and the observations then generalized to human behaviours, so it is open to criticism. Pavlov's and Skinner's work was based on the idea that if you repeated the same stimulus enough times and gave negative reinforcement (electric shock) or positive reinforcement (food) for incorrect and correct actions, respectively, eventually the subject would 'learn'. In an educational setting, their conclusions, which are the basis of behaviour theory or behaviourism, imply that the tutor or PE provides the negative or positive reinforcement of the behaviour to the learner. Reinforcement or punishment and reward continue to be explored in behaviour theory, although it is more politically correct to call them feedback, and to use positive rather than negative methods (Keck Fei et al. 2021). In ODP education, behaviour theory is relevant mainly to teaching clinical skills using simulations.

Clinical skills can be taught by breaking them down into steps, rehearsing each step, then the whole sequence, in a safe environment. Feedback is given to modify the behaviour. For example, if a learner scrubs in for the first time, but gets their scrubs soaking wet, the PE can modify that behaviour by demonstrating or suggesting another method that would keep them dry. The learner then adopts this behaviour as a result of the feedback (reinforcement) and reflects on their performance, successfully thereafter scrubbing in without getting wet (learning). This process can be seen in Kolb's cycle of experiential learning.

Behavioural objectives (see under 'Learning outcomes' later in this chapter) are very important in clinical training relating to operating department practice, especially as these objectives can be used as a guide for teaching and evaluating a learner's clinical performance. It can be argued that the foundation of perioperative practice education is behavioural competence (Aliakbari et al. 2015). Learning at the proficiency or mastery levels is explained by behaviours, and both of these derive from the expected learning outcomes of the curriculum and standards of proficiency for ODPs (HCPC 2017a and 2023; CODP 2018).

Cognitive theory

The theorists of the twentieth century believed that we learn by receiving information, processing it, storing it and then, later, retrieving it for use. Processing the information means you repeat it, use it, apply it and try a number of formats to see which work best. Learning comes from understanding, therefore the organization and structure of teaching contribute to learning. The discovery of knowledge or construction of meaning are also central to learning.

We can see cognitive theory in practice in a classroom setting, for example. You are given information, perhaps some individual problem-solving or group task that you work through with applied examples. The teaching is planned, organized and takes into account individual perceptions and differences (learning styles). You process the information, store it and, later, retrieve the information for use in an exam or discussion in practice. Another example would be a teaching session about the structure and function of the respiratory tract, disorders such as bronchitis, and the effects of disorders on its role in the activities of daily life. The students attending this session would come to understand the anatomy and physiology of the respiratory tract, a disease state (bronchitis) and the effects of disorders on the patient as a whole, not as three separate, unrelated topics (Aliakbari et al. 2015).

Cognitive feedback is an integral part of cognitive theory, similar to reinforcement in behaviourism. For example, your PE will provide you with constructive and organized feedback on your performance in practice. You will, hopefully, understand and identify your strengths and weaknesses and adapt your practice accordingly. Drawing on cognitive theory we can also examine the concepts of surface and deep learning approaches.

Surface learning

This type of learning is the storing of lots of information in the short-term memory for a specific purpose, such as for a written examination. It leads to the superficial retention of material (unprocessed) and does not promote understanding or the long-term retention of knowledge and information. To be able to understand and apply your learning, a deep learning approach is required.

Deep learning

This process involves the critical analysis of new ideas, linking them to concepts and principles you already know, and leads to the understanding and long-term retention of concepts, so they can be used for problem solving in unfamiliar situations (Advance HE 2020). It assumes that learning will be banked in your long-term memory as it has been learned, examined, considered, applied and understood. Table 1.2 summarizes the differences between surface and deep approaches to learning.

Stop and think

Looking at the characteristics listed in Table 1.2, can you identify your current approach to learning?

Think about the different elements of ODP professional knowledge. Do you, for example, see your knowledge of anatomy and physiology as separate from your anaesthetic, surgical and post-anaesthetic care knowledge?

Do you, instead, link all these aspects together to analyse patient care?

Table 1.2 The characteristics in surface and deep approaches to learning

Surface learning characteristics	Deep learning characteristics
• Relies on rote learning • Focuses on outward signs and the formulae needed to solve a problem • Receives information passively • Fails to distinguish principles from examples • Treats parts of modules and programmes as separate from one another • Does not recognize new material as building on previous work • Sees course content simply as material to be learned for an exam	• Looks for meaning • Focuses on the central argument or concepts needed to solve a problem • Interacts actively • Distinguishes between argument and evidence • Makes connections between different modules • Relates new and previous knowledge • Links course content to practice

Source: Adapted from Advance HE (2020)

Strategic learning

Strategic learning is when learners streamline their study to obtain higher grades and, hence, this approach is usually assessment driven. The effect is that they aim for a good grade without fully engaging with the depth and breadth of the content, so may forget the information as soon as they have passed that assessment. This approach is not beneficial to your development as a professional as it may result in the omission of key information, which could be to the detriment of your clinical knowledge and, ultimately, the quality of care you deliver.

Humanist learning

Humanist learning is student-centred and personalized, with the aim of developing self-actualized people in a co-operative, supportive environment. Humanist theory suggests that learning is a natural process and comes from within. Motivation, purpose and learning objectives are therefore important aspects that promote effective learning. However, they do not exist in isolation; you need to consider that you are an individual human being and various aspects of your life can affect your learning. A social or domestic situation, anxiety and emotion could all affect learning and your behaviour. For example, if you lack confidence in a particular situation, this may be exacerbated by stress in your personal life. However, the positive aspects of humanist theory are relevance and motivation, which you can use to help you. For example, being given responsibility aids learning, so a PE saying, 'You run today's operating list,' could allow you to develop your own skills and confidence.

Blended, remote and distance learning

The COVID-19 pandemic rapidly disrupted traditional modes of operation in healthcare and education. In response, the majority of universities and colleges in the UK had to change to make greater use of the digital delivery of course content. The terms 'blended learning', 'remote learning' and 'distance learning' came to be used more and more as a result. In this section, we explore the differences between these educational approaches and the skills that you will need to adapt to and get the most from them.

Blended learning

This type of learning provides face-to-face learning combined with dynamic digital activities and content that facilitate any time, anywhere learning. The balance between the classroom elements and digitally enabled activities will vary depending on the design and implementation of the learning by the educator. The flexibility integral to this form of delivery enables educators to rethink where and how they focus learning activities and allows learners to develop self-directed learning skills and digital literacy. An example of blended learning would be a session in which the facilitator introduces a clinical problem in a didactic form and then tasks groups or individuals with using library databases to identify current evidence-based practice that provides solutions to the problem. The content discovered would then be presented back to the class for discussion. You will find that this approach is commonly used as it engages learners in not only a clinical problem but also flexes their skills in relation to using digital technology, working collaboratively, appraising evidence-based practice and communicating to and with others.

This approach can be reversed, as in the example of a 'flipped classroom'. A flipped classroom is a pedagogical model in which the lecture and homework elements of a module or topic are reversed (Youhasan et al. 2021). Video lectures, texts or learning resources are viewed by learners at home before coming to the lecture. The lecture is then devoted to discussion and activities relating to the subject reviewed, so, in this example, a recorded lecture is seen as the key ingredient in the flipped approach. The video lectures can be developed by university educators or open education resources can be used. The lecture time is then facilitated by educators so learners can enquire about lecture content, test their skills in applying knowledge and interact with one another in hands-on activities.

Research demonstrates that blended learning, 'the mixing of online and face-to-face teaching, results in higher achievement, higher learner satisfaction, stronger learner persistence and larger flexibility in teaching and learning' (Thai et al. 2020).

Remote learning

This is a broad term encompassing any learning that happens outside the classroom, with the educator not present at the same location as the learner. Rapid developments in technology have made remote education easy. Most of the terms (such as online learning, open learning, web-based learning, computer-mediated learning and even blended learning) have in common the ability to use a computer connected to a network, which offers the possibility of learning from anywhere, any time, in any rhythm, with any means.

Remote learning methods and processes are really strong. They are learner-centred and offer a great deal of flexibility in terms of time and location. The COVID-19 pandemic saw an almost overnight shift to remote learning, enabling educators to adapt their teaching and processes to the needs of the learners. There are plenty of online tools available, which is important for an effective and efficient learning environment. Educators can use a combination of audio, video, text and virtual learning environments to reach out to their learners and, in times of crisis, do as much as possible to maintain a human touch in their lectures.

There are certain weaknesses inherent in remote learning, however. It can hamper aspects of communication between the learner and the educator, as it is not direct and so can feel as if you are disconnected. Users can face many technical difficulties and domestic distractions that can hinder and slow down the teaching–learning process (Dhawan 2020). Even before the pandemic, the literature uncovered several themes associated with student challenges to online teaching, including technological barriers, inadequacies in student–instructor communication and difficulties engaging students (Wallace et al. 2021).

As we learnt from exploring learning styles, learners are not all the same – they vary in terms of their capabilities and confidence levels. Also, not all learners feel comfortable learning online, which can potentially lead to increasing frustration and confusion. However, remote learning is likely to continue to be an integral component in HE in the future, in either synchronous or asynchronous form, and both educators and learners will need to carry on making the shift in their approach to teaching and learning from paper to pixels.

Distance learning

This form of learning, also referred to as 'online learning', is a common alternative route to studying for degree courses offered by universities and colleges. Instead of attending lectures and seminars on campus, the learner studies at home or work. The flexible and independent nature of distance learning often appeals to those whose circumstances prevent them from studying on campus, at a fixed pace, over several years. This might be due to them having a full-time job or other responsibilities, such as caring for dependents. Also, this enables international students to study remotely from their own country.

All teaching, materials and support are delivered online. Any assessments are done online, too, such as submitting assignments and, in some cases, taking examinations. A distance learning course is broken down into bitesize modules and learners can choose to mix and match different modules to attain the required credits for a degree. Distance learning has strengths and weaknesses similar to those of remote learning,

Some aspects of operating department practice can be taught by distance learning, but clinical practice cannot, for obvious reasons. Thus, distance learning is generally suited to courses with academic outcomes rather those required for a vocation, such as operating department practice, nursing and medicine, which require all the relevant standards of proficiency to be demonstrated in a registered healthcare professional (NMC and GMC 2021; HCPC 2023).

Skills needed to adapt to contemporary learning

To be successful when learning online, learners need both a set of generic skills and specific skills related to the digital platform that they will be using. For any one programme of study, there will be a diverse range of learners, experience and skills. The skills they will all need include the following (Sosulski and Bongiovanni 2013).

- **Digital skills:** At the very least, learners need to have basic computer skills to function effectively in a digital environment. You will be communicating with staff, practice educators and other learners through discussion forums, emails and video conferences or discussion boards. You may be uploading assignments, converting documents to PDF files and will need to be able to navigate within the course site and use the ePortfolio tool too.
- **Communication skills:** Depending on how the learning is presented, you may be communicating and collaborating with staff and peers in a variety of ways. Communication is usually either asynchronous, where learners post messages on discussion boards, for example, or synchronous, such as during a video session or in an interactive classroom.
- **Literature search skills:** You need to know how to use a variety of search tools to find scholarly articles, search databases, identify credible sources and locate primary and secondary sources.

- **Time management skills:** When online learning is used in conjunction with face-to-face learning, then deadlines are obvious. Where there is more flexible learning, however, the timings for study and so on are more self-directed and time management becomes even more important than usual.
- **Collaborative skills:** Working in small groups, sharing ideas and values, just as a learner would in a classroom setting but online, is very important. Research has identified that many students described feelings of loneliness and disconnect as they shifted from traditional to purely online learning environments. We are social creatures and we need human interaction. When collaborating on a project, therefore, you will need to develop your skills, listening to and depending on one other to generate new ideas. At the same time, you must also contribute.

Learning outcomes

Learning outcomes are the specified intended endpoints of a period of study activities. Ideally they should clearly indicate the nature or level of learning required to achieve them. They should also be achievable in a given timeframe and assessed by an appropriate method. The language used should be clear to learners, with explicit statements of what is expected of them, which will always contain verbs and other such words that express actions, events or expected behaviours (Quality Assurance Agency (QAA) 2007).

The use of learning outcomes is an integral part of the infrastructure of academic courses, deriving from curriculum competencies, subject benchmark statements and the framework for HE qualifications, which are integrated into programme and module specifications (CODP 2009; QAA 2018). Learning outcomes, both academic and clinical, are intended to enhance learning across a wide range of skills, which include the development of knowledge and understanding, cognitive/intellectual skills, as well as key transferable and practical skills. They provide information about the content to be learned and the way in which you will have to demonstrate that you have acquired satisfactory knowledge of it, enabling you to make appropriate choices about study methods and relevant content. Learning outcomes also facilitate the evaluation of your learning, as they are integral to the assessment process and criteria for assessment. For example, you can write and agree specific personal learning objectives with your PEs, to target and work on weaker areas of your practice. As a registered ODP, you can keep on setting learning outcomes to address your personal and continuing professional development (CPD) needs.

Individual learning outcomes may relate to the domains described in Bloom's taxonomy of the hierarchy of cognitive domains (Agarwal 2019), depending on the nature and what level of cognition (understanding) is being assessed. These may include the (Cassidy 2009):

- cognitive domain (knowledge and intellectual skills);
- psychomotor domain (physical skills, clinical practice);
- domain of professional behaviours (feelings and attitudes).

Table 1.3 Example of a clinical practice learning outcome

Learning outcome	Indicators of competency
Apply knowledge of pharmacology within operating department practice	Identify and demonstrate ability to supply appropriate drugs for use by the anaesthetist for **general** anaesthesia
	Identify and demonstrate ability to supply appropriate drugs for use by the anaesthetist for **regional** anaesthesia
	Apply local and national guidance/policies relating to the storage and checking of medicines
	Discuss the rationale relating to the selection of appropriate drugs
	An understanding of the pharmacokinetic and pharmacodynamic effects and contraindications of drugs used within the perioperative setting

During the course of learning, students will develop and attain different levels of cognitive, psychomotor and professional skills. Bloom originally identified six levels within the cognitive domain, from the simple recall or recognition of facts, as the lowest level, through increasingly more complex and abstract mental levels to the highest order, which was classified as evaluation (Bloom 1994). These levels can also be applied to the psychomotor and professional behaviour domains. Each domain has descriptions and associated verbs or statements that are often integrated into learning outcomes at different stages with educational programmes. Table 1.3 shows a clinical practice learning outcome used in operating department practice. To further define the skills or evidence required to meet the learning outcomes, as here, often indicators of competency are used (CODP 2018; HCPC 2023).

By setting clearly articulated learning outcomes/objectives, the ODP can develop metacognitive skills (knowing about knowing). These skills aid you in reflecting on and self-directing your thinking and learning processes. You can use your course's learning outcomes and clinical practice outcomes to monitor and evaluate your academic and clinical practice skills and progression. Ultimately, they will enable you to manage and develop your own learning more effectively.

Using mobile technology to aid learning

The use of information technology quickly became part of everyday life for most people in the Global North and is an integral part of university life and the learning process, too. Trends in mobile technologies suggest that they have the potential to have positive impacts on learning in general and HE in particular (Nikoi 2008; Sosulski and Bongiovanni 2013). As technology advances, there will be continued associated advances in the usability of mobile devices for teaching, learning and assessment. If you conduct a search of a device's applications available for download, the results will demonstrate how much educational material there is for learners. Potentially, learning may migrate to outside classrooms and lecture theatres and into learners' immediate environments (home or clinical placement) by means of mobile devices.

A number of educators already use micro-blogs to create a community around a class or an activity. Educators who have used X (formerly known as Twitter), for example, report that it is a useful feedback channel during and after class. After a lecture or seminar, tutors can encourage micro-blogging to support relationships between the people in the class and further their learning. Teachers post tips of the day, questions, information on writing assignments and other prompts to keep learning going. Another popular use of Twitter and micro-blogging sites is the building of professional networks. You can get to know other learning professionals, receive regular updates about professional practice, get help from experts and even attract followers of your own.

Here are some practical thoughts on how to make the most of mobile devices and IT when studying (adapted from the Open University 2022):

- set up reminders for tutorials or assignments on a calendar;
- create notes when you think of an idea for an assignment or a question to ask your tutor;
- record audio notes to summarize key points;
- check your facts on the web: try the library resources for your subject area, including websites, online journals and online books;
- download audio or video files to your mobile device;
- subscribe to podcasts and radio programmes related to the subject of your course;
- search the web for quizzes about your subject, so you can check your understanding;
- subscribe to really simple syndication (RSS) feeds of relevant information.

Recording lectures

When a learner believes that there are good academic reasons to request permission to record a lecture to support their learning, there will be a local policy that they will need to comply with. The recording of classes or clinical practice, and particularly sessions where patients and other learners are involved, is generally not permitted.

To fully realize the benefits of recordings *and* comply with the law, the HE institution must consider the rights of all relevant parties, including students, staff, patients and carers, whose work, participation and content may appear in an audio or video recording (Joint Information Systems Committee (JISC) 2010). Copyright and data protection law, under the Data Protection Act 1998 (2022), will be applicable where lectures, films, scripts, photographs, blogs and diagrams, for example, are being recorded. Also, a recording, as a work in its own right, will itself be protected by copyright. You should be aware, too, that professional and regulatory standards apply to all aspects of your conduct at university and should be adhered to at all times, especially in the context of recording lectures.

Since the COVID-19 pandemic, the availability of recorded lectures has increased exponentially (see under 'Remote learning', earlier in this chapter) and, hence, the need for learners to record lectures themselves has diminished. There is generally good availability of recorded remote learning material hosted in virtual learning environments.

Professional aspects of mobile technology

Learners must be courteous and respectful regarding the use of personal mobile devices in the classroom or a clinical placement setting. Furthermore, the growth and popularity of social networking websites makes it even more important for registered staff and learners to know how to use them without undermining their professional status. Ideally, social media can help learners to (HCPC 2017b):

- develop and share their skills and knowledge;
- help the public understand what they do;
- network with other professionals nationally and internationally;
- raise the profile of their profession.

Ly (2010) reported that it appears to be quite easy to blur the line between an individual's professional and personal life when using social networking websites. Commonly reported unprofessional postings include: violations of patient confidentiality, learners' use of profanity, discriminatory language, depiction of intoxication, and sexually suggestive material (Chretien et al. 2009; Ly 2010). As a response to these reported issues, universities, the HCPC (2017b) and employers have published clear guidance on the use of social media. Here are some of the HCPC's 'top tips' for using social media in ways that will not harm your professionalism.

- Think before you post. Assume that what you post could be shared and read by anyone.
- Think about who can see what you share and manage your privacy settings accordingly.
- Remember that privacy settings cannot guarantee that something you post will not be or not be made publicly visible.
- Maintain appropriate professional boundaries if you communicate with colleagues, service users or carers.
- Do not post information that could identify a service user unless you have their permission.
- Do not post inappropriate or offensive material. Use your professional judgement when deciding whether to post or share something.
- If you are employed, follow your employer's social media policy.
- When in doubt, get advice. Appropriate sources might include experienced colleagues, trade unions and professional bodies.

Simulation

With an increase in concerns for patient safety and the need to reduce critical errors in practice, ODP education continues to strive to develop competent and confident learners through formative learning experiences. Coupled with an increased knowledge of medical science, new treatments and complex healthcare systems, ODPs need to be capable of analysing a patient's clinical condition and responding accordingly, to implement safe and effective care (Reid-Searle et al. 2011). Consequently, the use of simulation, either formative or summative in nature, has evolved over the past 50 years from simple part-task training devices to complex mannequins, capable of imitating a variety of clinical situations (Harper and Eales-Reynolds 2011). Studies show that the use of simulation in an interprofessional context has a sustained, positive effect on learners' attitudes to learning and teamworking (Reid-Searle et al. 2011; Buckley et al. 2012).

Simulation can appeal to most learning styles as it enhances the cognition and psychomotor skills required to understand the clinical situation and the bigger concepts around collaborative working (Harper and Eales-Reynolds 2011; Buckley et al. 2012). Different complex situations can be created and analysed, but in a safe learning environment, promoting deep, reflective learning and the confidence to transfer new skills to the reality of clinical practice (Harper and Eales-Reynolds 2011).

The benefits of simulation are that it has intrinsic and extrinsic value for learners and, within universities, skills laboratories and simulation facilities provide valuable opportunities to enhance skills acquisition and they may be utilized to enhance clinical practice experience (CODP 2018). Importantly, simulation-based education offers the opportunity to practise or rehearse a wide range of skills to ensure that threshold standards are attained and retained. Simulation of practices can be particularly useful for rare clinical scenarios or those cases where students may not be able to fully participate in real situations, due to the safety and care needs of the patient.

Simulation has been proven to support the learning of skills in a safe environment prior to undertaking clinical placements. It can also be used to debrief students when experiential learning has presented challenges for them or where guaranteed safe, objective experience is not available. Research has identified that this approach has enhanced learners' skills application, cognition and confidence in performing various clinical tasks (Harper et al. 2016).

Stop and think

Reflect on an example of when you completed something in a simulation and in practice. How did the two experiences differ? Did you feel more prepared for the experience in practice following the simulation than you would have done without the simulation?

How do you think you could benefit from using your learning in both settings to support your future development as a learner?

Portfolios

The use of a portfolio is recognized as a valuable tool for the collection of evidence towards the assessment of the domains of practice (McColgan 2008) and should provide evidence of learning experiences and achievements in both academic and practice settings (Lewis 2010; Karsten 2012). Since 2009, ODP learners will generally each have a practice portfolio or ePortfolio that will contain, for example, academic achievements, practice outcomes, practice experiences, reflections and case studies (CODP 2018), thus preparing them for maintaining their evidence of professional development throughout their career. As information technology tools have been and continue to be developed and introduced into everyday life at university, it is important that the learner embraces and uses them. For example, the ePortfolio tool is an innovative and technically advanced method that can be used to demonstrate your academic achievements, clinical competences and critical thinking (JISC 2008; Lewis 2010; Karsten 2012).

The use of an ePortfolio has several benefits, which include:

- *demonstrating* improvements in the validity and reliability of practice assessment;
- the ability to link, inextricably, various sources of evidence to specific practice outcomes;
- the ability to reduce the amount of free writing for practice educators;
- the *improvement of feedback* between the learner and practice educator;
- *empowering* the learner to become self-reliant, organized and efficient in managing and recording their learning;
- integrating learning technology into the programme.

Learning support

Universities in England and Wales have a 'duty to make reasonable adjustments' for learners with disabilities, which includes learners with dyslexia or other specific learning needs. This duty of care ensures that individuals are not discriminated against in relation to 'the arrangements made for deciding upon whom to confer a qualification' under the Equality Act 2010 (Part 2, Chapter 1, Section 15).

Education providers have a duty to find out how they can make 'reasonable adjustments' to meet the needs of learners with disabilities. Whether an adjustment is reasonable depends on many factors, such as the cost of the adjustment – not only financially but also logistically – and its effect.

The intensity of ODP courses means that early diagnosis of learning disabilities is beneficial, so access to the screening of learners early on is common to ensure that individuals who need it are supported throughout their studies (Wray et al. 2008).

Revision strategies

Revising for an exam is one of the most individualized processes in academic life. There are many articles, books and advice on the subject of how to revise and

Table 1.4 An action plan for revision

Activity	Examples
Positive state of mind	Being motivated, positive messages, healthy lifestyle, accepting the challenge
Time	Engaging with revision early, organizing study time effectively, optimizing time, setting priorities
Variety	Study in short spells, use various techniques, make things interesting
Over-learning	Rewrite notes, make flash cards, essay, plans, creative trigger
Practice	Do past questions, engage with extended materials and set mock exam conditions
People	Share revision with others, have study buddies
Selection	What topics do I need to be revising? What level of detail do I need to include in my answers in the exam?

Source: Adapted from Burns and Sinfield (2012)

prepare for examinations. This chapter, therefore, provides insights and some useful guidance for ODP students.

The unique nature of ODP education means that students are often undertaking clinical practice while also preparing for exams, which can lead to stress for some learners. A little stress, however, can be positive and contribute to good psychological preparation. When experiencing too much physical or mental stress, however, the body increases its adrenaline levels, which gives rise to feelings of anxiety and tension, and these can have a negative impact on revision and exam performance (as described in humanist learning theory). Being fully prepared is generally considered the most effective way to overcome stress and anxiety about exams.

There are three revision strategies that have been shown to be useful to learners who have found traditional methods ineffective: being organized, using mind maps, creating a précis of your notes and using mobile technology.

Being organized

Burns and Sinfield (2012) suggest that having revision action plans adds discipline to your studies and ensures that you exploit and get control of your revision, thereby reducing stress. You should consider how the actions suggested in Table 1.4 can potentially help you when organizing your revision and preparing for exams.

Using mind maps

A mind map, or thought mapping, encourages the left and right hemispheres of the brain to integrate more, which, subsequently, improves memory. The left side of the brain is where the logical thinking occurs, whereas the right side has a more creative style. However, the brain uses both hemispheres to memorize information. The constructs of a mind map are ideally suited to encouraging both halves of the brain to work together more effectively and so make learning easier.

A mind map is a powerful non-linear (not like the text in this book) graphic technique that harnesses our full range of cortical skills, such as words, images, number, logic, rhythm, colour and spatial awareness. This is achieved in a single, uniquely influential manner and can give you an overview of a big subject or topic area. Mind maps can collect and hold large amounts of data and illustrate the links between different aspects of the topic. They also encourage active planning techniques because they allow you to see links and make connections in this way. It is visually stimulating and aids concentration and memory. Mind maps can be applied to any topic that you are studying, including planning essays, reports and presentations, as well as revision and note-taking tasks.

You can create your own maps quickly and effectively on a piece of A4 paper using coloured pens, but, if you prefer, there are software programs freely available in universities and the public domain that can create them for you. The use of colour, diagrams and images in mind mapping associates smaller bits of information and also encourages left- and right-side brain integration.

The value of creating a précis

Learners can often be under the illusion that every handout, textbook, article or web resource that is used on a course is equally important, so all of them must be read and integrated. Creating a précis, a synopsis or summary of your notes and materials, so your resources are more manageable, will make learning less stressful. Organizing information into a series of memory triggers, then reducing the number of triggers to a key word or image is a useful strategy. This can be done in the form of a mind map, with, for example, a central topic, then a branch and sub-branches. Generally, the advice is to learn the big things and summarize the smaller ones. The larger parts will act as rallying points to call the detailed abstract concepts to mind.

Mnemonics

These rallying points are memory triggers and need not be images. You can use a 'mnemonic', for example. 'Mnemonic' is another word for memory tool and is a technique for remembering information that is otherwise quite difficult to recall. A series of letters (an acronym) or words (usually a rhyme) are used as triggers for the recall of information, a process, sequences and so on. You probably remember the mnemonic for the colours of the rainbow. If you have just recalled it from, perhaps, your childhood, isn't that a good indicator of how useful they are? There are many medical mnemonics that learners can use to aid their recall of detailed information, such as 'To Zanzibar By Motor Car' for the five branches of the facial nerve – temporal, zygomatic, buccal, mandibular and cervical.

Stop and think

Mnemonics allow complex information to be condensed into an acronym or a few words, essentially making your memory more efficient. They are no substitute for hard work and wider reading, but that is of little use if you cannot recall your facts or get the information muddled up. Mnemonics allow you to secure information in your head with the aid of word play or visual associations.

Try creating mnemonics for:

- six functions of blood (factual exam revision);
- remembering the process for checking anaesthetic equipment (developing practice);
- the hierarchy of human needs (psychological theory).

Assessment

Assessment is a central component in the overall quality of teaching and learning in HE and should be viewed positively, as an opportunity to demonstrate the knowledge you have acquired. ODP courses may vary in how they assess academic and clinical skills. Most will use a mixture of assessment methods to capture an all-round, holistic view of a learner's competence and performance. Whether formative or summative in nature, however, assessment will always set clear expectations, establish a reasonable workload for learners and provide opportunities for you to self-monitor, practise and receive feedback. Assessment is an integral component of a coherent educational experience.

It is well documented that learners value, and expect, transparency in the way that their knowledge will be assessed. There needs to be a clear relationship between lectures, tutorials, clinical practice and subject resources and what they are expected to demonstrate in any assessment method used. Assessment is about making a decision regarding the present position of the learner's learning and, therefore, should be seen as a chance to consolidate your knowledge and understanding, in addition to demonstrating what you know to your tutors, PEs, patients and yourself (Burns and Sinfield 2012). Assessment can provide effective feedback about the grades achieved, reward your efforts and achievements and offer suggestions for how you can improve your all-round performance.

Summative assessment

Summative assessment is comprehensive in nature, provides accountability and is used to check the level of learning and experiences that have met the learning outcomes. This type of assessment is constructively aligned to reflect the learning outcomes (Biggs 2003; Burns and Sinfield 2012). For example, if on completion of a module you will have the knowledge and understanding to pass an exam, taking the exam would be summative in nature since it is based on the cumulative learning experience of the module. Summative assessments address the same domains, concepts and skills as formative assessments. They do not include anything new or unfamiliar to learners; the assessment has to be fair and valid (Cassidy 2009). Common summative assessment methods used in operating department practice education include assignments, examinations, presentations and the achievement of prescribed clinical practice outcomes.

It is important that an ODP learner understands the expected performance criteria (grading) in any summative assessment, as using the grades and the descriptor of the grades in formative assessment is a useful strategy when preparing for summative assessment. The ODP learner can then use these rubrics to self-assess their work formatively before finally submitting it to identify their academic strengths and weaknesses formatively.

Fotheringham (2010) provided a practical insight in the form of the concept of 'triangulation', supporting the use of multiple assessment tools. Using different methods provides a holistic view of academic performance, clinical skills and professionalism of the learner across the psychomotor, cognitive and professional domains (Gillespie and Hamlin 2009). PEs consider technical and procedural knowledge fundamental to clinical competence, but it must be acknowledged that communication, teamwork and co-ordinating the clinical workload are also important concepts that need to be included in the assessment process (Gillespie et al. 2009).

Grading competence

Perioperative competence is an eclectic concept that has been difficult to define and even more difficult to measure. Competence has been described in relation to standards of practice with little emphasis placed on its interpersonal aspects. Cassidy (2009) suggests that competence is something someone has learnt, giving them 'specialist' knowledge, characterized by familiarity with perioperative practice guidelines and standards of care, plus the human factors of interpersonal and social aspects of team interactions. However, there is no clear consensus on competence, and assessing a learner as competent may be complicated by the assessors' subjective interpretations of the assessment criteria (Cassidy 2009). Most literature on the subject of clinical competence advocates the use of rubrics or indicators to enable consistent assessment and evaluation of performance. Rubrics provide specific descriptions of the responses for each criteria and match proficiency levels and quality ratings. They precisely pinpoint what constituted the decision for the grade/scale given.

Competence grading scales and modified versions of them are often used in the assessment of clinical practice. Here, we reiterate the importance of formative assessment and effective, timely feedback (Juwah et al. 2004; Lennie and Juwah 2010). If both learner and PE use a scale, strengths and weaknesses across the practice domains can be identified and deficits developed further to meet the required grade. When learners engage with feedback, verbal or written, through reflective practice, new personal learning objectives can be set. If a learner failed a clinical practice assessment, for example, understanding the indicators used for the scale will enable them to identify criteria for development, but also provide justification for the assessment decisions made by the PE (Duffy 2003). The PE is seen as the 'gatekeeper' to the profession and has the professional responsibility of conferring competence on the learner – a decision that needs to be free from subjectivity (CODP 2009).

The issues of subjectivity and valid assessment for PEs contribute to the difficulties that they face when they need to fail a learner in clinical practice and, in some cases, they 'fail to fail' (Duffy 2003). The language used in assessment tools is an important factor in enabling the PE and learner to interpret competence (Gillespie et al. 2009). Competence assessment is affected by many situational factors, and Yanhua and Watson (2011) argue that these can detract from a valid, reliable measurement of the competence level of the learner. Furthermore, the clinical competence of newly registered staff has become a crucial issue in relation to profession standards and public safety (Darzi 2008).

It was professional behaviours and appropriate skills on the part of individual practitioners that were the overwhelmingly prevalent factors leading to the Mid Staffordshire NHS Foundation Trust public inquiry (Francis 2013). These professional values are central to the delivery of high-quality healthcare education and, therefore, PEs have a duty of care to the public, through their registrations, to ensure that learners develop into practitioners who are fit for purpose, to practise and to receive their award.

Formative assessment

Generally, formative assessment is designed to help tutors or PEs to identify learners' strengths and weaknesses through rich conversations that continually build and go deeper. It provides effective, timely feedback to enable learners to advance their learning and so actively involve them in their own learning. Ultimately, formative assessment nurtures in the learner the concept of increased autonomy and responsibility for learning (Andrade and Cizek 2010). The educational objective is to move the learner from being a passive receiver of information to becoming a self-reliant thinker (CODP 2018).

There are various methods that can be used in formative assessment, such as a logbook to record the number of orthopaedic cases you have scrubbed in for, to provide evidence of consistent practice. In more complex areas of practice, the use of high-fidelity simulations enables skills to be practised formatively in a safe environment and built on constructively before any holistic summative assessment is made. In an academic example, for an online quiz set by a tutor, a low score in pharmacology topics may indicate that there is a need to review the revision strategy or how the subject is learned. These examples identify strengths and weaknesses and, with feedback, enable learners to advance their learning in preparation for summative assessment.

Conclusion

The skills, practices and attitudes fundamental to being an ODP are gained from the whole educational experience. The information given in this chapter has provided a perceptive insight, for both new learners and those practitioners returning to learning, into the teaching, learning and assessment approaches used in the HE setting. It is hoped that the applied exploration of the topics covered in the course will contribute to a successful educational experience and lead you to become an autonomous, self-directed learner who is proficient in delivering evidence-based, individualized, high-quality patient care. Ultimately, developing your learning throughout your career as an ODP contributes to you becoming an accountable, responsible practitioner who is fit for purpose, practice and academic award.

Key points

- Understanding your learning style can guide you to success in your learning.
- Understanding educational theories helps to promote self-directed, self-reliant and effective learning.
- Understanding contemporary pedagogical approaches to teaching and learning.
- Use formative assessment as directive feedback to identify learning needs.
- Grading scales provide useful feedback and justify assessment decisions.
- A portfolio or ePortfolio is a valuable tool for the collection of evidence for the assessment of your practice and learning development.
- There are support mechanisms available for individuals with specific learning needs

---

References and further reading

Advance HE (2020) Deep and surface approaches to learning. York: Advance HE. Available at: www.advance-he.ac.uk/teaching-and-learning/curricula-development/education-mental-health-toolkit/learning-focused/deep-surface-learning (accessed September 2022).

Agarwal, P.K. (2019) Retrieval practice and Bloom's taxonomy: Do students need fact knowledge before higher order learning? *Journal of Educational Psychology*, 111(2): 189–209.

Aliakbari, F., Parvin, N., Heidari, M. and Haghani, F. (2015) Learning theories application in nursing education, *Journal of Education and Health Promotion*, 4: 2.

Andrade, H.L. and Cizek, G.J. (2010) *Handbook of Formative Assessment*. Abingdon: Routledge.

Biggs, J. (2003) Aligning teaching for constructing learning. York: Higher Education Academy (now known as Advance HE – name changed in 2018). Available at: https://s3.eu-west-2.amazonaws.com/assets.creode.advancehe-document-manager/documents/hea/private/resources/id477_aligning_teaching_for_constructing_learning_1568036613.pdf (accessed July 2023).

Bloom, B. (1994) Reflections on the development and use of the taxonomy, in Lorin W. Anderson and Lauren A. Sosniak (eds), *Bloom's Taxonomy: A Forty-Year Retrospective*. Chicago, IL: National Society for the Study of Education.

Buckley, S., Hensman, M., Thomas, S., et al. (2012) Developing interprofessional simulation in the undergraduate setting: Experience with five different professional groups, *Journal of Interprofessional Care*, 26: 362–9.

Burns, T. and Sinfield, S. (2012) *Essential Study Skills: The Complete Guide To Success At University*, 3rd edn. London: Sage.

Cassidy, S. (2009) Interpretation of competence in learner assessment, *Nursing Standard*, 23(18): 39–46.

Cherry, K. (2023) Overview of VARK learning styles. Verywell Mind. Available at: www.verywellmind.com/vark-learning-styles-2795156 (accessed July 2023).

Chretien, K.C., Grevsen, S.R., Chretien, J.P. and Kind, T. (2009) Online posting of unprofessional content by medical students, *Journal of the American Medical Association*, 302(12): 1309–15.

College of Operating Department Practitioners (CODP) (2009) Standards, recommendations and guidance for mentors and practice placements: Supporting pre-registration education in operating department practice. London: CODP.

College of Operating Department Practitioners (CODP) (2018) Bachelor of Science (Hons) in Operating Department Practice – England, Northern Ireland and Wales; Bachelor of Science in Operating Department Practice – Scotland: Curriculum document. London: CODP.

D'Amore, A., James, S. and Mitchell, E.K.L. (2011) Learning styles of first-year undergraduate nursing and midwifery students: A cross-sectional survey utilising the Kolb Learning Style Inventory, *Nurse Education Today*, 32(5): 506–15.

Darzi, A. (2008) High quality care for all: NHS next stage review final report. CM 7432. London: Department of Health (DH).

Dhawan S. (2020) Online learning: A panacea in the time of COVID-19 crisis, *Journal of Educational Technology Systems*, 49(1).

Duffy, K. (2003) Failing students: A qualitative study of factors that influence the decisions regarding the assessment of students' competence in practice. Glasgow: Caledonian Nursing and Midwifery Research Centre, Glasgow Caledonian University.

Fotheringham, D. (2010) Triangulation for the assessment of clinical nursing skills: A review of theory, use and methodology, *International Journal of Nursing Studies*, 47(3): 386–91.

Francis, R. (2013) Report of the Mid Staffordshire NHS Foundation Trust public inquiry: Executive summary. HC 947. London: The Stationery Office. Available at: https://assets.publishing.service.gov.uk/government/uploads/system/uploads/attachment_data/file/279124/0947.pdf (accessed September 2022).

Gillespie, B.M., Chaboyer, W., Wallis, M., et al. (2009) Operating theatre nurses' perceptions of competence: A focus group study, *Journal of Advanced Nursing*, 65(5): 1019–28.

Gillespie, B.M. and Hamlin, L. (2009) A synthesis of the literature on competence as it applies to perioperative nursing, *Association of Perioperative Registered Nurses*, 90(2): 245–58.

Harper, M. and Eales-Reynolds, L.J. (2011) Simulation: Knowledge transfer from classroom to patient care, *Technic*, 2(4): 12–15.

Harper, M., Markham, C. and Givati, A. (2016) A pilot study of Operating Department Practitioners undertaking high-risk learning: A comparison of experiential, part-task and hifidelity simulation teaching methods, *Journal of Pedagogic Development*, 6(2): 58–65.

Health and Care Professions Council (HCPC) (2017a) Standards of education and training. London: HCPC.

Health and Care Professions Council (HCPC) (2017b) Guidance on social media. London: HCPC.

Health and Care Professions Council (HCPC) (2023) Standards of proficiency: Operating department practitioners. London: HCPC.

Horton, D., Wiederman, S. and Saint, D. (2012) Assessment outcome is weakly correlated with lecture attendance: Influence of learning style and use of alternative materials, *Advances in Physiology Education*, 36(2): 108–15.

Hydrie, M., Naqvi, S., Alam, S.N., et al. (2021) Kolb's learning style inventory 4.0 and its association with traditional and problem-based learning teaching methodologies in medical students, *Pakistan Journal of Medical Sciences*, 37(1): 146–50.

Joint Information Systems Committee (JISC) (2008) Effective practice with e-Portfolios. Bristol: JISC Infonet.

Joint Information Systems Committee (JISC) (2010) Recording lectures: Legal considerations. Bristol: JISC Legal Information.

Juwah, C., Macfarlane-Dick, D., Matthew, B., et al. (2004) *Enhancing student learning through effective formative feedback*. York: HEA Generic Centre.

Karsten, K. (2012) Using ePortfolio to demonstrate competence in associate degree nursing learners, *Teaching and Learning in Nursing*, 7: 23–6.

Keck Frei, A., Kocher, M. and Bieri Buschor, C. (2021) Second-career teachers' workplace, *Journal of Workplace Learning*, 33(5): 348–60.

Kolb, D.A. (1984) *Experiential learning: Experience as the source of learning and development*. Upper Saddle River, NJ: Prentice Hall.

Kurt, S. (2022) Kolb's experiential learning theory and learning styles. Educational Technology, 25 September. Available at: https://educationaltechnology.net/kolbs-experiential-learning-theory-learning-styles (accessed July 2023).

Lennie, S.C. and Juwah, C. (2010) Exploring assessment for learning during dietetic practice placements, *Journal of Human Nutrition and Dietetics*, 23: 217–23.

Lewis, T. (2010) Working measures: Online clinical practice assessment, *Technic*, 1(2): 15.

Ly, K. (2010) Social networking: Blurring the personal and professional, *Technic*, 1(18),: 2–3.

McColgan, K. (2008) The value of portfolio building and the registered nurse: A review of the literature: Karen McColgan explores the value of portfolio building, *Journal of Perioperative Practice*, 18(2): 64–9.

Nikoi, S. (2008) *Work-based Learners in Further Education (WoLF) Project*. Leicester: University of Leicester.

Nursing and Midwifery Council and General Medical Council (NMC and GMC) (2021) Joint statement on professional values. London: NMC and GMC. Available at: www.nmc.org.uk/news/news-and-updates/joint-statement-from-chief-executives-of-statutory-regulators-of-health-and-social-care-professionals (accessed September 2022).

Open University (2022) Study skills for online learning. London: Open University. Available at: https://help.open.ac.uk/browse/study-skills/study-skills-for-online-learning (accessed September 2022).

Quality Assurance Agency (QAA) for Higher Education (2007) *Outcomes from Institutional Audit: The Adoption and Use of LEARNING Outcomes*. Gloucester: QAA.

Quality Assurance Agency (QAA) for Higher Education (2018) Quality code. Gloucester: QAA. Available at: www.qaa.ac.uk/quality-code (accessed September 2022).

Reid-Searle, K., Eaton, A., Vieth, L., et al. (2011) The educator inside the patient: Learners' insight into the use of high fidelity silicone patient simulation, *Journal of Clinical Nursing*, 20: 2752–60.

Rohrer, D. and Pashler, H. (2012) Learning styles: Where is the evidence?, *Medical Education*, 46: 630–5.

Sarafino, E.P. (2008) *Health Psychology: Biopsychosocial Interactions*. Hoboken, NJ: John Wiley.

Sosulski, K. and Bongiovanni, T. (2013) *The Savvy Student's Guide to Online Learning*. New York: Routledge.

Thai, N.T.T., De Wever, B. and Valcke, M. (2020) Face-to-face, blended, flipped, or online learning environment?: Impact on learning performance and student cognitions, *Journal of Computer Assisted Learning*, 36(3): 397–411.

Wallace, S., Schuler, M.S., Kaulback, M., et al. (2021) Nursing student experiences of remote learning during the COVID-19 pandemic, *Nursing Forum*, 56(3): 1–7.

Wray, J., Harrison, P., Aspland, J., et al. (2008) The impact of specific learning difficulties (SpLD) on the progression and retention of learner nurses. Hull: University of Hull.

Yanhua, C. and Watson, R. (2011) A review of clinical competence assessment in nursing, *Nurse Education Today*, 31(8): 832–6.

Youhasan, P., Chen, Y., Lyndon, M., et al. (2021). Exploring the pedagogical design features of the flipped classroom in undergraduate nursing education: A systematic review, *BMC nursing*, 20(1): 50.

Further reading

Legislation

Data Protection Act 1998: www.legislation.gov.uk/ukpga/1998/29/contents (accessed September 2022).

Equality Act 2010: www.legislation.gov.uk/ukpga/2010/15/contents (accessed September 2022).

2 Evidence-based practice, research, audit and service evaluation for operating department practice

Hannah Abbott

Key topics

- The origins and development of professional knowledge
- Evidence-based practice
- Research
- Research ethics
- Paradigms of research
- Quantitative research
- Qualitative research
- Mixed methods research
- Literature review
- Critical appraisal of literature
- Clinical audit
- Service evaluation

Introduction

As Operating Department Practitioners (ODPs), we use research evidence throughout our careers to develop our knowledge and enhance our practice. It is therefore important to understand how this knowledge is generated so that published research can be critiqued and used effectively to inform practice. This chapter explores the philosophy that underpins research and the methodologies that may be employed in healthcare research. As research is an extensive topic, it is not possible to cover all aspects in depth within this chapter. The main aim here, therefore, is to provide an overview of the principles of research and clinical audit that will give you the skills you need so you can read and appraise published research effectively, thus enabling you to utilize evidence in your career as an ODP. The other aims are to demonstrate that research is integral to the professional role of ODP and give you the confidence to consider your own research interests and how you may develop these further.

Why is this relevant?

There are many national publications relating to different aspects of healthcare delivery. However, all of them have one key theme: the delivery of high-quality patient care. The responsibility for delivering this care is shared by all practitioners.

As ODPs, how do we know that we are delivering high-quality care to every patient and we are instilling this culture in all we do in our professional practice?

Ultimately, we have to start with our own individual practice and ODPs must 'be able to assure the quality of their practice' (Health and Care Professions Council (HCPC) 2023: Standard 11), which includes engaging in evidence-based practice, the systematic evaluation of practice and seeing the value of data for quality assurance/improvement and to evaluate patient feedback (HCPC 2023). It is therefore considered impossible for an ODP to deliver high-quality care and meet the threshold standards for professional registration without engaging with research.

The perioperative environment is a dynamic one that is continually evolving to meet increasingly complex needs. These may be the patients' needs and the complexity of the co-morbidities or they may be to do with the delivery of anaesthesia or complex surgical procedures and equipment. Whatever the nature of the complexity, the knowledge and skill set of ODPs must advance so that we can meet these needs, and ODPs therefore need to engage with research, as it is part of their professional responsibility to do so: 'you must keep your professional knowledge and skills up to date and relevant to your scope of practice' (HCPC 2016: 7). This may be achieved in a number of ways as part of continuing professional development (CPD), which is discussed in more detail in Chapter 11. However, it is not possible to ensure that our knowledge is current without ever reading about the new developments, so do take a look at research published in a range of journals, accessible via a National Health Service (NHS) OpenAthens account or university databases.

In addition to contributing to the ODP-specific body of knowledge, ODPs are one of the Allied Health Professions (AHPs) and so have an important contribution to make to growing the collective body of AHP research too. The 'Allied Health Professions research and innovation strategy for England' was published on 26 January 2022 and covers the totality of the AHP workforce in recognition of the need to increase the pace of growth of AHP research and innovation (HEE 2022). This strategy identifies an ambitious vision for transformational change in the approach to research, which is intended to support and enable new and exciting opportunities for ODPs' engagement with research.

This chapter therefore supports you in your endeavours to engage with research to provide high-quality care and for your own development as a professional.

The origins and development of professional knowledge

Think about our professional practice for a moment. Why do we do things in the way that we do? For example, why do you lay your scrub trolley out in a certain way? Maybe it is because that is how you have always done it, maybe it is how you were taught by your practice educator or maybe it is your 'hospital's way'. A lot of the skills we have were taught to us by practice educators, who were taught by practice educators before them, but how did that knowledge originate and how did it evolve?

As mentioned, some of the operating department practices have been passed from ODPs to students over the years, through teaching, observation of practice and via textbooks, and this is termed 'traditional knowledge'. This knowledge is considered important in terms of both the necessity to share and learn it, and in its role in the development of ODPs' professional identity (Parahoo 2014). Some of these traditional practices become rituals that are performed without thinking about them in an analytical way but, rather, simply carried out as they always have been (Courtney et al. 2010). It has been suggested that ritualistic practice helps practitioners and patients to manage the emotional and social interactions that are involved with the role (Strange 2001). It is not acceptable, however, to simply undertake tasks automatically without ever questioning how they are done. This is not to say that some of these traditional practices are suboptimal – it may be that what we are doing remains the best approach – but to validate this, we must question and explore the evidence.

Professional knowledge has itself also evolved through a process of experience and reflective practice (see Chapter 5) and the results of experiential learning then and now can be shared to enhance the learning experiences of others. While experiential learning is valuable in perioperative practice, it is important for ODPs to also recognize that this knowledge will be limited by their own experiences and so we must be aware that relying purely on experiential knowledge can, in fact, restrict our professional development. For example, an ODP working with paediatric patients may feel that one distraction technique is preferable for cannulation as this has always worked effectively for them and their colleagues in the past. However, this historic local practice may restrict further development as the ODPs may not be willing to explore new techniques and so miss ways to improve on the current practice.

Linked to experiential learning is the consideration of intuition as a source of knowledge. However, this is difficult to define and cannot be the topic of empirical research (Parahoo 2014). Despite this, many ODPs may report having 'a feeling' that something is wrong or requires further investigation. It may be argued that such a feeling is not intuition but, rather, the result of a combination of clinical knowledge, experience and systematic patient assessment that allows a practitioner to rapidly assimilate information regarding the patient and make a prompt decision regarding the care plan.

Professional knowledge is forever evolving and while some of our current practices may be attributed to tradition, ritual or experiential learning, this is clearly not sufficient to ensure that the provision of care continues to be of a high quality. This is not to suggest that current perioperative practice is poor; rather, it should be questioned to ensure that it truly is the best current practice, based on robust evidence.

Stop and think

How confident do you feel about explaining the evidence base underpinning your practice?

Would you be able to refer to literature? Could you explain the alternative methods and show why yours is best overall?

For example, if someone asked you, 'Why do you assist with rapid sequence induction in that way?' how would you answer? Because it was the way you were taught, it is what the anaesthetist concerned prefers or would you be able to discuss and critique the literature regarding the efficacy of cricoid pressure, the amount of pressure and the timing of its application?

Remember that registered ODPs must 'be able to practise as an autonomous professional' (HCPC 2023: Standard 4), which requires ODPs to be able to justify their decisions.

Evidence-based practice

In this chapter so far, we have considered the evolution of our professional knowledge and why we need to be able to provide a rationale for our practice that is based on evidence. This leads us on to the principle of evidence-based practice.

There are misconceptions about evidence-based practice, such as that by following the recommendations of one published paper, an ODP is implementing evidence-based practice. However, it is not that, nor is it practising in a traditional, ritualistic way because that is how you were taught some time ago (Prasun 2013). The term 'evidence-based practice' means having a focus on empirical evidence for what is effective in practice (Glasziou et al. 2003) and therefore involves integrating research evidence with clinical experience and knowledge of a patient or a procedure in the context of the patient's own preferences and values (Sackett et al. 2001). In short, the ODP needs to be able to assimilate all the necessary knowledge related to a case and use this to inform their practice accordingly. For example, the ODP may consider the empirical knowledge about the benefits and limitations of spinal anaesthesia in conjunction with knowledge gained from a qualitative paper about the patient experience and use these together with their own clinical experience and assessment of the patient to deliver an evidence-based plan of care to that perioperative patient.

Evidence-based practice is implemented on a larger scale by means of evidence-based practice guidelines. These are developed by synthesizing the evidence and considering its validity to make recommendations for practice (Beyea 2004). It is considered that once these guidelines have been implemented, this should reduce variability and result in an overall improvement in patient care (Beyea 2004). It is important, however, for clinical guidelines to be reviewed on a regular basis, as new research findings may mean that they need to be updated to ensure practice continues to reflect the most current, valid evidence base.

Research

Research is a systematic process that generates new knowledge to contribute to a wider body of knowledge. The 'body of knowledge' is a phrase that is used often to describe the knowledge that is unique to a specific topic area. Hence, the operating department practice body of knowledge includes clinical practice and knowledge specific to the education of ODPs. The ODP-specific body of knowledge is evolving as more practitioners undertake research and publish their findings in professional journals, something that is key to the development of our profession. Some aspects of our body of knowledge overlap the body of knowledge of associated professions within the perioperative environment and, hence, there are opportunities for collaborative research projects across all disciplines in the field of perioperative care.

There are differing views regarding the purpose and application of research. The traditional, scientific view of research is that it is purely for the discovery of important knowledge rather than the application of this knowledge, and hence it has been argued that researchers are not responsible for the impact or application of their research. Many ODPs and other healthcare practitioners may find that this traditional view conflicts with their professional obligations for their activities to be of benefit to patients. However, there is also the view that those who fund research have an influence on the objectives and potential applications of the study. In the case of publicly funded research, it has been suggested that the public (our potential patients) should have a role in the identification of research priorities. Thus, if we consider research in the context of the perioperative environment, it would seem crucial that the research is relevant to the service provided and has some benefit to patients, and so, while healthcare research does contribute to the body of knowledge, it is also designed to make a contribution to professional practice.

Aims, questions and hypotheses

All research projects will have a clear focus, but depending on the topic and approach, this can be expressed in a number of different ways – as an aim, a question or a hypothesis. It is important to note that while a researcher will establish this early in their research, it may not be explicitly stated in the published paper, but it will be evident from the title and introduction.

Setting an aim for a research project allows the researcher to express a statement of intent and provides a focus for the study. This is often used in qualitative research that takes a more reflexive approach. When stating an aim, it needs to be achievable within the bounds of the study, such as, 'the aim of this study is to determine patients' lived experience of day surgery'.

Framing the study topic as a question is another common approach, and it can be used effectively for quantitative and qualitative primary research as well as literature review projects. Asking a question in this way is particularly useful for new researchers as it provides a clear focus – the study must answer the question. In healthcare research, a PICO framework is often used to define the question – that is, it considers the population, intervention, comparison and outcome. An example would be, 'Does total intravenous anaesthesia (intervention) reduce the incidence of post-operative nausea and vomiting (PONV) (outcome) when compared with sevoflurane (comparison) in adult patients undergoing gynaecological surgery (population)?'. Using this framework can be helpful in refining an initial research idea into a clearly focused question, as it allows the ODP to narrow the focus of their study and the process encourages the consideration of variables that can have an impact on the results and how they can be reduced by clearly focusing on the population to be studied. The PICO framework is also frequently used to frame the questions for literature reviews and the process can then be used to support the identification of search terms, as multiple terms can be identified under each section. There are limitations to this tool, however, as, in some studies (particularly qualitative ones), there may not be a defined outcome or, in others, there may not be a comparison and so, while the principles may be helpful, it is important that PICO is used as an enabling tool rather than a restrictive one.

Hypotheses are commonly employed in quantitative studies and form a key component of statistical analysis. A 'hypothesis' is simply an educated prediction of the expected findings; this may result from previous studies or a review of the literature. The key to using a hypothesis to express the study focus is that the hypothesis must be testable and the study should seek to prove or disprove the overarching hypothesis. Consequently, this is the usual approach taken for scientific, experimental studies. In quantitative research, inferential statistical tests are performed under the null hypothesis (discussed later in this chapter).

Research ethics

It is essential that research has robust governance mechanisms to ensure high standards of research and ethical practice. The 'UK policy framework for health and social care research' replaces previous governance frameworks and sets out the principles of good ethical practice to follow when conducting research (NHS Health Research Authority (NHS HRA) 2021a).

Research ethics is a complex topic and the underpinning principles of ethical practice are explored in more detail in Chapter 9, so in this chapter, the aim is to provide you with an overview of the practical considerations regarding research ethics. The primary consideration for any research must be the protection of the participants' dignity, rights, safety and well-being and, consequently, informed consent is central to ethical research (DH 2009). To ensure informed consent has been obtained, all potential participants must be fully informed about the risks, benefits and potential discomfort related to participation, the aims of the study, its methodology, sources of funding and their right to withdraw at any time. It has been shown that patients' satisfaction with the information provided to them in studies could be improved (Länsimies-Antikainen et al. 2009) and, hence, it is good practice for participants to be given written information as a point of reference. This may be prior to data collection, so that a patient has sufficient time to consider their participation properly prior to their surgery.

In the UK, ethical approval for healthcare research is sought via the NHS Health Research Authority's Research Ethics Service (NHS HRA 2021b). It aims to protect the interests of research participants and to facilitate ethical research that has benefits for both the participants and the wider community. Research proposals are submitted to Research Ethics Committees (RECs), which are independent panels that review applications and decide whether the proposed research is ethical

(NHS HRA 2021b; see website for more details of the application process). It is essential that ethical approval is obtained prior to commencing data collection and, consequently, the time needed to complete this process must be factored into any work plan. In the case of research that is undertaken as part of a university programme of study and does not involve data collection in a hospital, such as a project to determine the knowledge other healthcare students have of the ODP role, ethical approval must be obtained from the university's ethics committee instead. In addition to gaining ethical approval, appropriate access permissions must be sought from the individual or organization responsible for the 'care' of the participants. Note that it is not appropriate to collect data from any participants without this approval.

Paradigms of research

A 'paradigm' is a philosophical belief system and, in the context of research, this is the fundamental belief regarding the production of knowledge. In research there are two differing belief systems regarding the generation of knowledge and these translate into two approaches to research: quantitative and qualitative. It is often assumed that these two approaches are themselves defined by the variable measured and whether this is a quantity or a quality, but that is not the case. Rather, it is the underpinning philosophy that defines the methodology. It is possible, therefore, to measure a quality (for example, feelings of satisfaction), but using a quantitative approach that results in numerical data for analysis.

In the positivist paradigm, the belief is that objective knowledge can be produced by employing a rigorous methodology (Broom and Willis 2007) and so the scientific method of testing a hypothesis and using a reductionist approach to reduce phenomena to statements of law based on the probability of their occurrence is used (Parahoo 2014). The positivist approach therefore underpins quantitative research, which uses scientific principles to produce firm conclusions and 'rules' relating to perioperative care that can be generalized to the wider population. An example would be the efficacy of different anaesthetic agents.

Interpretivism is in direct contrast to positivism, the view being that knowledge is a social construct, and so, to understand human behaviour, it must be explored in the context in which it occurs (Parahoo 2014). This philosophical approach therefore underpins qualitative research, which explores lived human experiences and behaviours in specific settings, so offers greater depth, but the results cannot be generalized in the same way that they can for quantitative research. Therefore, using interpretivism to explore ODP students' experiences of their clinical placements, for example, would produce results that were specific to the hospital placement (context) and may not be generalized to all ODP students, who would undertake placements in different contexts, such as specialist hospitals.

Quantitative research

'Quantitative research' uses numerical analysis to examine the relationships between measured variables. For example, an ODP may use this approach to determine if there is a relationship between the duration of an anaesthetic and the length of time spent in the post-anaesthetic care unit. Quantitative research, therefore, can provide important information that will have a direct impact on the care of patients. For example, research into the efficacy of a procedure when compared with an alternative or the incidence of side effects for a particular drug. Consequently, the findings from such research can have a direct impact on the care of perioperative patients and the provision of services in a department.

Methods

There are different quantitative methodologies that may be employed to address a research question, but generally these can be described as one of three different designs: experimental, survey or case study.

- **Experimental research designs** are aimed at determining the relationships between variables, and a range of experimental methodologies may be employed to do this. The 'randomized control study' (RCT) is considered the most robust methodology as participants are assigned randomly to either an intervention or a control group. The effect of the intervention can then be determined by comparing the results for the two groups. The RCT design is generally used when trialling a new intervention. Quasi-experimental studies also compare the effect of an intervention against a control group, but the participants are allocated to the two groups rather than randomized. This type of design is also used for before and after studies, which are frequently used to measure the efficacy of healthcare interventions (Centre for Reviews and Dissemination (CRD) 2009).
- **Survey research designs** are used to collect a large amount of information from a population. This approach is commonly employed by ODPs conducting research to improve practice in the perioperative environment. This approach can collect information regarding the incidence, frequency, severity and distribution of variables within a population, which can then be examined to identify relationships within the data. This approach would have been used to identify the risk factors for PONV mentioned earlier in this section, by surveying the patients who experience this, the nature of their surgery, their age and gender.
- **Case studies** focus on specific situations and involve collecting a range of information pertinent to the given subject of the study. This data will be predominantly descriptive, although researchers do explore any relationships between the variables (Parahoo 2014). ODPs may use this approach, at a local or national level, to explore a specific adverse incident, such as difficult airways.

These are the most frequently employed approaches to research design, but there are other specific methodologies within these categories. Also, there is some potential for methodologies to be adapted to fit specific topics. When undertaking research as part of an academic award, the paradigm and design are aspects that you would discuss with your supervisor.

Blinding

Blinding may be utilized in quantitative studies to minimize the risk of observer bias as, theoretically, if either the participant or the observer knows which group they have been allocated to, it may have an impact on their responses . There are two types of blinding.

- **Single blind studies**, in which either participants or researchers (not both) do not know the group allocation arrangements – they are 'blind' as to which group they are in. In single blind studies, it is generally the participants who are blind as to whether they are in an intervention or a control group. An example might be when a patient does not know which anaesthetic maintenance agent they are receiving.
- **Double blind studies**, in which both the participants and the researchers are blind.

When you read research papers, the methodology will often include blinding and how this was achieved. It is necessary, therefore, to consider how important blinding is to the results. For example, objective physiological measurements will not be affected by knowledge of group allocation. Any safety considerations of blinding must also be considered, such as a situation in which the patient and/or the researcher did not know the nature of the medication administered. In addition, there are potentially ethical issues related to blinding. For example, when 'sham surgery' is used for the control group, consideration would need to be given to whether it is ethical to subject participants to an unnecessary anaesthetic (Katz 2006).

Sampling

When collecting data for quantitative studies, ideally the ODP researcher would like to collect data from everyone in the relevant population. However, this is not feasible and so it is necessary to collect data from a sample of the relevant population.

There are several different sampling methods that are commonly employed in quantitative research. These are usually probability samples that are randomized by, for example, using computer-generated random numbers or random number tables. There are also non-probability sampling methods that are occasionally employed, such as for accidental or volunteer sampling, which are samples of convenience. However, these approaches do not have the same rigour as randomized techniques as not all members of the potential population have an equal chance of being selected, hence bias can be introduced at this stage of the study. For example, if you wanted to discover what the public know about the role of ODPs, you could survey passers-by in a town centre one weekday. However, this would exclude a large proportion of the working population and, thus, introduce bias. It is important that ODPs undertaking research consider how they will identify their sample and it is useful to read a number of papers to see what methods other researchers have used effectively to collect data in the perioperative environment.

The sample size is also central to quantitative studies as it must be sufficiently large to detect any significant differences , but it is not appropriate to collect excessive amounts and unnecessary data. Thus, the sample size is generally determined by a 'power analysis'. This is a calculation that considers the magnitude of the expected difference due to the intervention to give the number of participants required to show a statistically significant difference, if one exists. If the expected difference is small, then a larger sample size will be required to show any significant differences. It should be remembered that some studies will conduct their power analysis based on the primary outcome, so they may be underpowered for any secondary outcomes. ODPs should therefore also consider the sample size in the context of their clinical knowledge to assess what will be adequate for the purposes of the research and the feasibility of collecting the data in the given time.

Data collection

Quantitative data can be collected in a number of ways to meet the aims of the study. This frequently involves collecting experimental data or physiological measurements.

Many quantitative studies that aim to gain information about the patient experience will use surveys. These may include simple 'yes or no' questions or more complex scales to grade the information provided. Many ODPs use surveys in their research as these are an effective way to gather a large amount of data. However, the response rates tend to be low and so a significant number of questionnaires need to be distributed to elicit the required number of responses. The development of surveys is a complex process and, hence, sufficient time must be allocated for this and to test the survey instrument for 'construct validity', which means to test that the survey measures what it is intended to measure.

Data analysis and statistics

The statistical analysis of data is a feature of quantitative research studies and can be found in the results section of a published paper. There are two types of statistical analysis: descriptive statistics and inferential statistics. It is important for ODPs to have an appreciation of both types if they are to be able to appraise a paper critically and effectively.

'Descriptive statistics' feature in all quantitative papers and are also used when reporting clinical audit results. These serve to summarize and describe the data using simple mathematical measurements, such as the mean value, the range and percentages. They also allow you to compare the results for two sample groups, so you may, for example, read that there is a higher incidence of anti-emetic therapy following isoflurane maintenance (38.1 per cent) than when propofol is given (11.9 per cent; Gecaj-Gashi et al. 2010). While you can see any observed differences between the two groups, you may also want to know whether the difference is a true difference, resulting from the interventions, or it may have occurred by chance. It is in such cases that inferential statistics are beneficial.

'Inferential statistics' also feature in the majority of quantitative research papers but are not generally used in clinical audit. These statistics are used to determine whether the observed relationship is greater than that which would be expected by chance and, hence, whether it is a true relationship between the two variables or it has occurred by chance (Katz 2006). There are several statistical tests that can be performed (see Table 2.1) on the data and which one is used will depend on the type of data, whether the test aims to determine difference or correlation or whether the data is parametric. 'Parametric data' is normally distributed and, hence, most biological measurements result in normally distributed data. Table 2.1 is designed to serve as a point of reference when reading published

Table 2.1 A summary of commonly used statistical tests

Statistical tests	Tests for . . .	Data
t-test	Differences between two population means	Parametric
Mann–Whitney U test	Differences between two population medians	Non-parametric
Wilcoxon matched-pairs (signed-rank) test	Differences between population medians of two matched samples or compare before and after results	Non-parametric
Analysis of variance (ANOVA) test	Difference between population means of more than two populations	Parametric
Kruskal–Wallis test	Difference in medians of three or more populations	Non-parametric
Pearson correlation coefficient	Correlation between two data sets	Parametric
Spearman's rank correlation coefficient	Correlation between two sets of measurements	Non-parametric
Chi-squared (or chi-square) test	Association between two variables	Non-parametric

papers and conducting a critical appraisal of them, as this process asks you to consider the suitability of the statistical tests employed.

All these statistical tests are performed under what is known as the 'null hypothesis', which means that there is no difference/correlation/association (as appropriate to the test) between the two (or more) variables. The statistical test is then performed to determine whether the null hypothesis can be rejected or must be accepted based on the critical probability (p-value) of 0.05. A calculated probability of less than 0.05 ($p < 0.05$) is considered statistically significant and so allows for the rejection of the null hypothesis and, thus, the acceptance of the alternative hypothesis, which is that there is a statistically significant difference/correlation/association between the variables. In the study by Gecaj-Gashi et al. (2010) mentioned earlier in this chapter, a p-value of 0.011 was calculated, which is less than 0.05 and so the null hypothesis, that there is no significant difference, could be rejected. This meant it could be concluded that there is a significant difference in the incidence of anti-emetic therapy dependent on whether isoflurane or propofol anaesthesia was given.

The calculation of such probability values is generally carried out using specific statistical software and, where it has been used, the names and versions will be mentioned in the research papers.

It is important to become familiar with these tests. ODPs need to be able to consider descriptive and inferential statistics discussed in research results if they are to make valid judgements as to the significance of the findings from research for practice.

Qualitative research

'Qualitative research methods explore people's subjective experiences and opinions in order to better understand and give meaning to social phenomena' (Appleton 2009: 20). Consequently, qualitative research is highly valuable for operating department practice, as we may seek to determine patients' lived experiences of a particular procedure or event. Typically, the data produced during the course of qualitative studies is rich and highly relevant to practitioners, especially as ODPs tend not to receive detailed feedback from patients about their experiences in the perioperative environment.

Methods

Qualitative researchers aim to explore experiences and to do this generally use one of three main approaches.

- **Ethnography** is rooted in anthropology and so behaviour is explored in the context of the setting in which it occurs. This may be particularly valuable for ODPs as it is recognized that the perioperative environment is a unique one. For example, an ethnographic approach, using observation and interviews, could be used to explore the behaviour of parents accompanying children into the anaesthetic room.
- **Phenomenology** explores peoples' perceptions and lived experiences. An ODP could use this approach to gain rich data related to patients or students in the perioperative environment, such as patients' experiences of an unscheduled Caesarian section and the care they received.
- **Grounded theory** develops theories from social research data and, hence, differs from many methods, which generally use data to verify theories (Glaser and Strauss 1967). Grounded theory is a commonly used technique for developing ODPs' understanding of patients' experiences. Such studies generally use interviews to collect data from people who have undergone a specific procedure or care in a specific environment (such as day surgery) and this is then used to develop theories and hypotheses.

Sampling

Qualitative research is concerned with gaining detailed information about very specific experiences and, therefore, data is collected from a relatively small sample of participants (generally fewer than ten). Consequently, ODPs conducting this kind of research will need to select participants who are suited to the study's aim. Generally, therefore, a purposive sampling technique is adopted so participants selected can provide the required information.

Data collection and analysis

The aim of qualitative research is to collect detailed data and, hence, ODP researchers need to select a tool that elicits in-depth information. Consequently, interviews and focus groups are a common method of data collection for such studies.

Interviews can be approached in a variety of different ways – they can be structured or semi-structured, for example. Researchers need to identify which option will be the most appropriate for their study. Data is usually collected by making audio recordings that are later transcribed for analysis. It is often considered beneficial for researchers to transcribe their own recordings, so they become familiar with the data and can listen to differences in vocal expression. The analysis of this qualitative data is complex and generally involves identifying themes. Coding and triangulation may also be used. Hence, it is important to consider how the data is to be analysed and discuss this with a supervisor well before commencing a qualitative study.

Mixed methods research

Mixed methods research is becoming increasingly recognized as a valuable methodology. This is particularly the case in healthcare research where often we want to understand the scale of the issue as well as the patient experience, so a mixture of methods enables us to take advantage of both quantitative and qualitative approaches to provide the data needed (Östlund et al. 2011).

It may be argued that the term 'mixed methods' also relates to studies that combine two qualitative or two quantitative methods, which is known as 'within paradigm research' (Morse 2010). For example, an ODP may want to research surgical site infection (SSI) and, therefore, may want to collect data regarding the incidence and severity of SSI (quantitative), but also find out what the patients' experience of this is (which could be quantitative, by using a survey, or qualitative, via patient inverviews, for example).

There are various definitions of mixed methods research and there is often some overlap with a 'multiple methods' approach, which is when two research projects are included within the same study. However, it has been recognized that a true mixed methods approach has a primary philosophical approach with a secondary approach that explores this further (Driessnack et al. 2007; Morse 2010). A mixed methods design, therefore, 'consists of a complete method (i.e. the core component), plus one (or more) incomplete method(s) (i.e. the supplementary component[s]) that cannot be published alone, within a single study' (Morse and Niehaus 2009: 9). Therefore, in the example of an ODP researching SSI, the quantitative method (collecting objective data) would be the primary approach and the exploration of the patient experience would form the secondary, qualitative approach.

The validity of this mixed methods approach to research has been widely debated, but it is considered to be a pragmatic approach (Mendlinger and Cwikel 2008) that is particularly useful in healthcare research because of the complexity of the research questions posed in this field (Östlund et al. 2011). In addition to the complexity of the research questions, funding bodies have also expressed a preference for healthcare research that uses different methods for data collection and considers aspects of both biomedical and social science (Tritter 2007).

There are several methodological approaches to mixed methods studies that are commonly employed (Tritter 2007).

- **Quantitative + qualitative**, which starts with a quantitative study that initially collects data – the frequency of a phenomenon or biological/physiological data, for example. Then there is a second phase, which uses a qualitative approach to explore the experience of the individuals concerned in depth. For example, an ODP may use this approach to explore PONV, as in the first stage, a large-scale quantitative approach could be used to collect data about the incidence, severity and treatment of PONV, then in the second, qualitative stage, the patient experience and the impact of the different options on recovery could be explored through an interview approach.

- **Qualitative + quantitative**, which uses a qualitative approach initially, to identify key themes, and these then inform the development of the data collection tool for the larger-scale quantitative component. This approach could be employed, for example, to determine the student experience of pre-registration ODP education by conducting some initial interviews or focus groups, then using the key themes that emerged from these to produce a questionnaire that would be circulated to a large number of ODP students.

- **Qualitative + qualitative (QUAL + qual)**, which uses a standard qualitative method as the primary method for gathering data (such as phenomenology, ethnography, grounded theory), and then supplements this with a component from another qualitative method, such as focus groups or observation (Morse 2010).

The analysis and reporting of results from mixed methods studies is challenging and it has been shown that a separate analysis of the quantitative and qualitative data is common. In addition, there is often a lack of clarity as to whether the reported results originate from the quantitative component or the qualitative one (Östlund et al. 2011). It has been suggested that triangulation should be employed to analyse the multiple data sets as this process is believed to produce a stronger conclusion when the results are convergent, but this will not always be the case and the two methods may report disparate results (Al-Hamdan and Anthony 2010). When planning a mixed methods study, therefore, ODPs should consider the options for data analysis early in the process and discuss them with their supervisor as investing this time and thought early on in the project will enhance the work overall.

Mixed methods research, then, is an evolving approach to perioperative research that can result in valuable information. However, as a developing approach, it presents a number of challenges regarding the combining of two distinctly different paradigms and the resulting data analysis. It is essential, therefore, that these elements are clearly described in the paper and the origins of the results are also clearly presented (Östlund et al. 2011). Despite these challenges, mixed methods research has the potential to make valuable contributions to the body of ODP knowledge.

Literature review

Literature reviews are a highly valuable contribution to evidence-based practice as they require the author to collate, summarize and critically discuss the key information about a chosen topic. They also form the first stage of a primary research project, as it is necessary to review what is already known about a topic before starting a primary research project.

The process of conducting literature reviews is important for all ODPs, both in the development of our own practice and for the purpose of advancing our profession by undertaking them for publication in professional journals. Reading published literature reviews is also valuable for ODPs as they each provide an analytical review of a chosen topic that allows you to get a good understanding of current research, which can be used to inform our own practice.

Narrative review

Narrative reviews are the most straightforward type of literature review and are similar in format and process to some academic assignments. You will find some published in journals that provide a broad review of a particular topic. The aim of a narrative review is to illustrate the development of concepts, theories and methods in an area. The review will therefore synthesize and discuss the previous research and consider it in the current context and the context in which the original literature was produced, to interpret the information correctly (Jones 2007). The nature of a narrative review, however, is that it does not follow a strict process for identifying and selecting which articles to include, nor do those articles undergo a rigorous appraisal process. For these reasons, narrative reviews are most commonly used by ODPs to update their knowledge rather than to inform or change practice.

Systematic review

'Systematic reviews seek to collate evidence that fits pre-specified eligibility criteria in order to answer a specific research question. They aim to minimize bias by using explicit, systematic methods documented in advance with a protocol' (Cumpston et al. 2023). A systematic review, therefore, involves taking a robust approach to a literature review, which is important when the findings are to be used to inform professional or clinical practice. Cochrane (n.d) is a global organization with a mission to produce 'trusted synthesized evidence' to inform health decisions. There are more than 7,500 systematic reviews in the Cochrane Library, so it is a good place to start when looking for examples of systematic reviews. In addition, the Cochrane Library has published resources relating to systematic reviews that can be found online.

A systematic review should be as exhaustive as possible to minimize the risk of failing to identify relevant studies (CRD 2009). Therefore, ODPs should search a full range of journal databases, which are accessible via university e-resources or via an NHS Athens account. In addition, ODPs will need to perform a citation search, to identify any potentially relevant papers that have not been found in the initial searches. While this search may identify a number of relevant papers, the nature of it prevents the identification of recent papers, as they cannot be cited in older publications (CRD 2009), so this needs to be considered in the context of the study. Google Scholar may be a useful resource, as it includes a range of publication formats, including peer-reviewed papers (Bell 2005), and while it may not be possible to obtain the full text for every article, these can generally be ordered via university or hospital libraries.

When starting a systematic review, generally a low-precision, high-yield search using key words is the first step. However, such a search will result in a considerable number of results, so it will then be necessary to reduce this yield by using a high-precision, low-yield strategy (Smith and Dixon 2009). It is at this point that Boolean operators are used to combine relevant terms to narrow the search. Records of this need to be kept as a summary of the process followed needs to be included in the published article or completed work as the research protocol.

Once a number of studies have been obtained, the papers are selected in accordance with strict inclusion and exclusion criteria appropriate to the research question. For example, an ODP may consider it appropriate to include only in-patients or patients over the age of 18. Alternatively, emergency cases may be excluded if the focus of the review is elective procedures.

Stop and think

Imagine that you wanted to explore post-operative recovery after a laparotomy as a research project.

- What search terms would you use? How many different words might be relevant to recovery? Would you include pain, analgesia (as there would be a require-ment for more analgesia if pain scores were high), PONV or sickness among your terms?
- Who would you include or exclude? Would you want to exclude emergency sur-gery (if so, what category?), as then patients may have had less pre-operative optimization?

There is no absolute right or wrong answer. Simply make sure that the papers you find are relevant to the research question and you can justify the inclusion and exclusion criteria.

The papers selected for inclusion then undergo a rigorous critical appraisal process to assess their validity and reliability. It is considered good practice to have a minimum of two researchers appraising the papers independently and agreeing the results to reduce subjectivity, bias and error (CRD 2009; Parahoo 2014). However, this is not possible when conducting a systematic review as part of a university programme of study.

Following this appraisal, the researcher will identify key themes in the litera-ture and undertake a critical analysis of these that will form the main body of the systematic review. This critical analysis will synthesize the data presented in the selected papers and the quality of these studies. Identifying relationships between findings, considering the impact of any methodological limitations and noting areas for further research will be addressed in the discussion. To aid this reporting of systematic reviews the 'Preferred Reporting Items for Systematic Reviews and Meta-Analyses (PRISMA) statement' may be beneficial. This is an evidence-based, 27-item checklist that clearly sets out the minimum requirements for reporting a systematic review. While it is primarily designed for reporting reviews evaluating the effectiveness of interventions, it can also be used for sys-tematic reviews with other objectives (PRISMA 2021).

While systematic reviews are of existing published literature, they themselves are subject to critical appraisal. They may vary in quality due to either the methodology or the quality of the studies included. Methodological limitations may be the result of bias introduced by the researcher. For this reason, ODPs must be aware that published systematic reviews should still be read critically.

Systematic reviews typically include only peer-reviewed papers, but this results in publication bias within the study, as the only research considered is that which has been published in academic journals. To eliminate publication bias it is necessary to compare published data with unpublished studies (CRD 2009). However, locating suitable unpublished data can be challenging and such studies may not have been subject to the same quality assurance procedures as the published ones, such as ethical approval or peer review. Further, many systematic reviews include only articles written in English, which introduces a language bias because research with statistically significant results is more likely to be published in English-language journals than research that does not have significant results, leading to a potential bias in the conclusions (CRD 2009).

There are some practical considerations that can be followed to avoid bias. For example, best practice for systematic reviews is to include all potentially relevant research, irrespective of the language of the publication. This does present some difficulties for ODP researchers, but they should be able to justify decisions made regarding inclusion and recognize the potential impact on their work.

Systematic reviews offer ODPs a good opportunity to engage with and undertake a research project without the requirement for ethical approval and, hence, are generally a more easily accessible option. Depending on the context of the project, a team can be established and, therefore, there may also be opportunities to work with more experienced researchers, which will serve to develop your skills and confidence in this process. It is also good to discuss your ideas with ODP colleagues who have completed a systematic review as part of a previous project as this will help you to refine your own thinking.

Critical appraisal of literature

Purpose

A critical appraisal of literature is a process that is directly connected to the use of a literature review as a research methodology, but being able to appraise work critically is an important skill for all ODPs to possess and apply more generally, as it is invaluable when reading research papers or other publications to assess their true value. This is because there is considerable variation in the quality of research studies and any methodological limitations that introduce bias can have a significant impact on the results. Being able to make a critical assessment of the quality of a study allows you to determine whether the results can be 'believed' and are sufficiently reliable to be used to inform practice (CRD 2009). In addition, the nature of the online environment means that the majority of ODPs have access to a considerable amount of information and this, too, varies in quality and accuracy, so it is important that the skill of critical appraisal is developed and applied. This process is discussed further later in this section.

Stop and think

When you read journal articles or other published material (especially online), do you accept it as being best practice? Or do you seek to consider the strengths and limitations of the information by, for example, questioning the methodology and the validity of the results?

Sometimes people feel that they cannot question published literature as it has been published by reputable organizations or journals and/or are written by individuals who may be more academically qualified than they are. This is not the case, however, as all ODPs should question the quality of the information they are using to inform their practice. It is also important to consider how applicable any findings are in the context of your own practice area. It is even more important to apply your critical reading skills to the other published material available online, which is not necessarily subject to any formal peer review process.

Principles

The measure of quality is often considered a subjective measure, but the CRD (2009) has defined some guiding principles to follow when assessing the quality of a research study.

- The suitability of the study design in terms of meeting the research objective(s) must be considered. If the design chosen for the study is inappropriate, then there is little value in continuing with the appraisal.
- The risk of bias must also be considered, which may be the impact a number of methodological decisions have, such as those relating to blinding or sampling. The general principle regarding bias is that a study must seek to control for any variables that could influence the results. For example, in the study regarding PONV discussed earlier in this chapter, the sample size chosen and sampling strategy would seek to result in two study groups that did not have any demographic differences, as it is known that females have a higher incidence of PONV and, therefore, if one group had a significantly more female participants than the other, this would introduce a bias.
- The selection of outcome measure(s) must be appropriate as that is how the efficacy of the intervention will be measured. In quantitative studies, this is particularly important as it is directly connected to sample size when a power analysis is performed.
- The statistical tests performed must be considered in terms of their suitability for use with the data and in relation to the study's objectives, in addition to examining the results obtained. The statistical significance reported should also be considered in the context of the observed differences, as there may be a clear observed difference that is not statistically significant, which may suggest that either the sample size was too small or further research is required.
- The quality of the intervention should be examined, as there may be anomalies in how it was performed or it may be so different from your own practice area that the results may not be applicable to your own practice.

- The quality of the way the study is reported in the paper must be examined for clarity – is it clear how the study was conducted and what the results are?
- The final consideration is the generalizability of the findings, in terms of the wider population and different practice settings. This is also when, as an ODP, you will consider the applicability of the study to your own practice area, so it is important to think about how the context of the research environment may have had an impact on the results.

Tools

There are tools that can be used to guide the critical appraisal process and it is worth spending some time becoming familiar with these to see which ones you find easiest to use. Some of the commonly used tools are listed below, but there are others available, so the list should not be considered prescriptive but, rather, be used as a starting point.

- The **Critical Appraisal Skills Programme (CASP)** tools are frequently used by ODPs as they were designed to support evidence-based practice in healthcare by encouraging the development of skills in a location, appraisal and utilization of evidence in healthcare decision-making. There are several different CASP checklists available and ones specific to different types of studies (RCT, systematic reviews and qualitative studies, for example), which can be downloaded from CASP's website (CASP 2021).
- The **LoBiondo-Wood and Haber** (2006) guidelines are very detailed and explicitly consider a number of potential threats to the validity of a study. The quantitative tool is particularly suited to the appraisal of papers aiming to test a hypothesis, and ODPs may find them especially useful when appraising laboratory-based studies (such as in drug research).
- The **Litva and Jacoby** (2007) tool is designed specifically for the appraisal of qualitative research and, therefore, the questions are focused on key aspects of qualitative methodology (such as triangulation).

These tools are designed for published research or literature review articles, but it is important to apply robust skills of critical appraisal to other publications that do not conform to a standard research paper format. ODPs should also remember that these tools are purely to aid and guide the process and it is possible to appraise a paper critically without using any tools. Indeed, as you become more familiar with the process, you will find that reliance on these tools will decrease.

In addition to research papers, ODPs are used to using clinical guidelines to inform their own practice on a daily basis, and these guidelines are also subject to scrutiny and critical appraisal, as 'the potential benefits of guidelines are only as good as the quality of the guidelines themselves' (AGREE Next Steps Consortium 2017: 1). Therefore, you may want to appraise a guideline either for your own practice or because you are developing a new or similar guideline for your own clinical area. The Appraisal of Guidelines for Research and Evaluation II (AGREE) is an international tool for healthcare practitioners to critique guidelines. It also aids the development of guidelines by providing a process for this and a guide for the inclusion and presentation of information (AGREE Next Steps Consortium 2017). These processes are highly relevant for ODPs as the skills of critical thinking and appraisal need to be transferable to all areas of practice. Also, understanding the process of guideline development enables you to appreciate how research can be used to inform and enhance patient care on a large scale.

Stop and think

Why not try reading a journal article using this questioning/critical approach? You might want to download one of the CASP tools to help you or you can simply consider the research in the context of everything you have read in this chapter. Alternatively, you may prefer to use highlighting or annotate the article to identify its strengths and limitations.

Having done this, how has reading the article in this way had an impact on your practice? Or do you not consider the article of sufficient quality to affect your practice – is further research needed?

Now consider how you can use this process as part of your CPD.

Clinical audit

'Clinical audit' is defined as 'a quality improvement cycle that involves measurement of the effectiveness of healthcare against agreed and proven standards for high quality, and taking action to bring practice in line with these standards so as to improve the quality of care and health outcomes' (HQIP 2020: 4) 'Audit' is distinctly different from 'research', but the preparation for and execution of clinical audit work will employ a number of the principles and skills required for research, which is why it has been included in this chapter.

Clinical audit may be undertaken at two levels: national and local. National clinical audits are large-scale projects that assess compliance with standards on a national level by collecting data submitted by healthcare providers. An example of this is the National Clinical Audit and Patient Outcomes Programme (NCAPOP), managed by the Healthcare Quality Improvement Partnership (HQIP). NCAPOP includes more than 30 national audits to develop a national view of the care standards for 30 common conditions (NHS England n.d.). The aim of national audits is to influence the development of national standards and processes and, hence, will result in an impact at local level (Bullivant and Corbett-Nolan 2010). A greater number of ODPs, however, will contribute to local-level audits that measure performance in one hospital or department, or even in one specific operating theatre, depending on the topic.

Audit is a key component of clinical governance, as the continuous improvement of services can be directly facilitated by the clinical audit process (Grainger 2010). Consequently, the importance of clinical audit to governance and service delivery should be recognized by NHS boards as being key to monitoring the efficacy of hospital strategies to delivering improvements (Bullivant and Corbett-Nolan 2010). However, it must be recognized that, while important, clinical audit is one element in any quality improvement strategy and so it is key to also consider whether it is the most appropriate mechanism to meet the specific needs or aims in each situation (Bullivant et al. 2015).

The explicit relationship between clinical audit and improvements in services resulted in the recognition that the subject clinical audit must be embedded in the education of ODPs to equip them with the confidence and skills needed to engage with the process (Bowie et al. 2010). This was achieved, clinical audit for ODPs having featured in the pre-registration curriculum for some years (College of Operating Department Practitioners (CODP) 2006, 2011, 2018) and, indeed, this subject contributes to the requirement for ODPs to 'assure the quality of their practice' (HCPC 2023). Despite this, there may be ODPs who feel that they need to update their skills in this area and, while there are several ways to do this, it is advisable to contact the local hospital's audit department first, as it may offer training sessions or be able to direct ODPs to audit work currently being under-taken, so it may be possible to gain experience of working with a team on an audit and then progress to leading an audit.

In addition to the need to develop the necessary skills, additional barriers to undertaking and implementing audit within the NHS have been identified. Research has shown that practitioners report pressures of work and lack of protected time as barriers to engaging in audits (Bowie et al. 2010) and, therefore, it is important that this is considered at the planning stage and discussed with managers.

Stop and think

How often do you think, 'I wonder if we, as a department or profession, are con-sistently following best practice?'

Or maybe you think, 'Our practice is really good, but do I have any evidence to support this?'

This could become a topic for clinical audit and, if so, ask yourself, 'How confident would I be about planning and implementing audit? Do I need to develop my knowledge and skills further?'

Differences between audit and research

The primary focus of clinical audit is on the improvement of practice, which is unlike research as its primary purpose is to contribute to the body of knowledge. While it could be argued that research may also result in improvements to prac-tice, this is not the fundamental reason for undertaking research.

The audit process is focused on current clinical practice, and making observa-tions and comparisons between this and best practice, hence, ethical approval is not required. However, audits should be registered with the relevant hospital's clinical governance department, in accordance with any local policy. Although formal ethical approval is not required, there are ethical and legal issues that relate to the audit process. For example, the standards of conduct, performance and ethics (HCPC 2016) needs to be adhered to throughout and, if patients are asked to comment on any aspect of the care provided, you need to ensure they are aware that the (anonymized) information may be shared to support improvement of the service (Patel 2010).

Stages and process

Clinical audit follows a set process or cycle that consists of four stages (HQIP 2020). This has been reduced from the five stages previously advocated by the National Institute for Health and Clinical Excellence (NICE 2002).

- **Stage 1: Preparation and planning.** This stage of clinical audit is crucial and, hence, it is important that sufficient time is spent on it. Once the purpose of audit has been clearly identified, the audit team can be established. It is important to consider the skills and expertise that will be required to produce a successful audit. For example, you may require representation from a surgical ward or feel that you need someone with expertise in data analysis. The team can then plan the audit and will need to develop a structure and work plan together that includes regular team meetings. While this may be challenging, it is essential to the success of the project. One of the defining characteristics of clinical audit is the use of explicit criteria and standards, against which performance is measured and, hence, these must be established and based on the best available evidence, which needs to be referenced (HQIP 2020). At this stage, all governance arrangements must be established alongside preparing to collect data in accordance with data protection legislation.
- **Stage 2: Measuring performance.** Measuring the level of performance is a significant part of the process and so a significant amount of careful planning is required for it. This applies particularly to the tools developed for and then used to collect the data for analysis. Clinical audit may be either prospective or retrospective, and which approach you choose will influence how you develop the tools to be used so that they are appropriate. Both approaches have strengths and limitations, therefore, the team needs to consider which is most suited to the topic and will provide the required data most effectively. The data collection tool is then developed and, as is essential to ensuring the success or otherwise of the audit, it should include 'relevant, concise and unambiguous questions' (Grainger 2010: 32). For some audit topics relating to national guidelines, there are set audit tools available, which should be used, so whether this is the case for your topic should be confirmed prior to starting to develop your own. When this has been done, the data is then collected throughout the audit period from the agreed sample of patients, selected based on inclusion or exclusion criteria that have been set beforehand (NICE 2002). The data is then analysed and the results compared with the criteria and standards. It is essential that the clinical audit method is recorded in detail so a future repeat of the audit can be completed in exactly the same way (HQIP 2020).
- **Stage 3: Implementing change.** Clinical audit is a quality improvement process and, therefore, once the results have been analysed, it is essential to develop an action plan to implement improvements and for this to focus on any areas of practice that led to a poor outcome in audit (Copeland 2005). The actions required will depend on the results of audit but, typically, these involve

staff education and training and possibly the introduction or a revision of systems of practice through changes to local or national policy (Ashmore and Ruthven 2008). One such action may be for ODPs to deliver additional training or write or update a departmental policy.

*   **Stage 4: Sustaining improvement.** This is the final stage of clinical audit process as, having completed the work involved in the audit process itself, it is important that it then results in a sustained improvement in practice. While it may be argued that it is the responsibility of individual perioperative practitioners to follow the outcomes of changes to processes, it is also important that the originating team ensures these are monitored and, hence, it is usual for there to be a follow-up audit after three to six months. In addition to following up with another audit, continued activities to promote awareness of and engagement with the changes made may be beneficial to the ongoing improvement in services. It is also essential that the outcomes of audit and action plan are shared, with the stakeholder group, service users and more widely across the organization (HQIP 2020).

Service evaluation

To 'assure the quality of their practice' (HCPC 2023), ODPs may elect to undertake a service evaluation, either as part of an academic award or their ongoing clinical work and professional development. While this requires the use of some of the research skills discussed so far in this chapter, it is a distinctly different activity.

A 'service evaluation' is undertaken to 'describe and investigate the efficiency of an established service or clinical intervention with the purpose of generating information that is of local significance. The aim of a service evaluation is to generate information that can be used to inform local decision-making' (Brain et al. 2011: 22). This definition is important as the fundamental aim of a service evaluation is to evaluate an existing service at a local level, unlike research that generates new knowledge to be used to introduce, change or improve a service or practice and be applied more widely. The other key difference is that the evaluation does not change the standard service delivery and the participants will be those normally using that service (King's Health Partners 2022), and their care is planned and delivered independently of the service evaluation (NHS HRA 2022). Hence, the service evaluation does not change the planned care and, as such, typically uses existing data, although it is possible to include interviews or questionnaires (NHS HRA 2022). Also, as a service evaluation is not research, it does not require approval from a research ethics committee (NHS HRA 2022) but, prior to commencing, advice should be sought regarding the local governance arrangements that apply to the service evaluation, both in the clinical organization and in the university concerned, if the service evaluation is part of an academic award.

When planning a service evaluation, typically practitioners will follow a five-step 'evaluation cycle' process, as advocated in the NHS and partners' (n.d.) Evaluation Works Toolkit.

*   **Step 1: Identify and understand.** In this stage, it is key to develop an understanding of the service to be evaluated. This will include exploring the evidence

and any literature related to the service, identifying the stakeholders and local experts.

- **Step 2: Assess.** This stage includes assessing whether there is a need for an evaluation, the potential benefits and that the resources that will be required are justifiable. It is also important to assess that the planned project is a service evaluation and not research – this is key as it can be easy to stray into research, which has different ethical requirements.
- **Step 3: Plan.** During this stage, the detail of the evaluation is planned, including the aims and objectives, the data required and how this will be collected.
- **Step 4: Do.** It is in this stage that the data is collected and analysed.
- **Step 5: Review and act.** This stage involves the review of the data to collect and interpret the findings. These can then be disseminated and there are a number of ways this may be achieved: via local presentations, reports, leaflets or more creatively, in the form of an infographic, for example. Finally, the results of the evaluation can be used to make evidence-based recommendations for practice and an action plan to implement these.

Stop and think

All the different approaches covered in this chapter will enable you to find ways to improve the quality of your practice and service delivery. The important thing is to select the correct approach for your project. For example, if you wanted to explore mandatory training for ODPs you could:

- undertake a service evaluation to ask ODPs how well they think their existing mandatory training is delivered;
- carry out audit to compare the completion and pass rates for mandatory training against the standard set by best practice;
- organize a research project to identify the most effective delivery methods for training to determine which is the best approach to maximize knowledge retention following mandatory training.

Now think about an area of practice you are interested in. How could you make it the focus of a service evaluation? Or audit? Or a research project?

Conclusion

The aim of this chapter has been to review key principles related to research and ODPs and, hopefully, it has contextualized some key concepts for you. It is sometimes believed that, to conduct research, you need to have completed postgraduate study, or research is only ever conducted as part of a formal academic award. It is hoped this chapter has demonstrated that is not the case and there are several ways in which ODPs can become engaged in research. Research is rarely undertaken in a solitary manner and, therefore, if you feel that this is an area you want to develop, you may want to see what opportunities there are to engage with projects at your place of work or study, or in collaboration with others in the Allied Health Professions, as this will help to develop your knowledge and skills as a researcher.

It is important that, as an ODP, you recognize engaging with research is part of your role and profession, and reading research papers is essential to ensure your professional knowledge is current and you are part of delivering the best care to our patients. As you progress through your career as an ODP, it is important to continue to question your practice and that of others and address this by reading the literature or maybe undertaking your own research project, as it is only by doing this that our practice and our profession will continue to develop.

Key points

- Engaging with research to deliver evidence-based care is an essential part of the professional role of an ODP.
- The aim of research is to contribute to the body of knowledge, but, for health-care practitioners, there is an additional aim, which is to improve patient care and service delivery.
- There are two distinctly different overarching philosophical standpoints that have defined the paradigms of research, resulting in the two main approaches: quantitative and qualitative.
- Literature reviews are important for the development of professional knowledge and are frequently conducted to inform and set standards for practice.
- It is essential for ODPs to develop the skill of critical appraisal so that they are able to review information in a critical manner to assess whether it is valuable and pertinent to their practice setting.
- Clinical audit is a key component of clinical governance and is used to review practice against set standards and make improvements. By contrast, a service evaluation measures an existing service but does not measure it against a standard.

References and further reading

AGREE Next Steps Consortium (2017) AGREE II Instrument. Agree Trust. Available at: www.agreetrust.org/resource-centre/agree-ii (accessed January 2022).

Al-Hamdan, Z. and Anthony, D. (2010) Deciding on a mixed-methods design in doctoral study, *Nurse Researcher*, 18(1): 45–56.

Appleton, J.V. (2009) Starting a new research project, in J. Neale (ed.), *Research Methods for Health and Social Care*. Basingstoke: Palgrave Macmillan.

Ashmore, S. and Ruthven, T. (2008) Clinical audit: A guide, *Nursing Management*, 15(1): 18–22.

Bell, J. (2005) *Doing Your Research Project*, 4th edn. Maidenhead: Open University Press.

Beyea, S.C. (2004) Evidence-based practice in perioperative nursing, *American Journal of Infection Control*, 32: 97–100.

Bowie, P., Bradley, N.A. and Rushmer, R. (2010) Clinical audit and quality improvement: Time for a rethink? *Journal of Evolution in Clinical Practice*, 18: 42–8.

Brain, J., Schofield, J., Gerrish, K., et al. (2011) A guide for clinical audit, research and service review: An educational toolkit designed to help staff differentiate between clinical audit, research and service review activities, rev. edn. London: Healthcare Quality Improvement Partnership. Available at: www.hqip.org.uk/wp-content/uploads/2018/02/hqip-guide-for-clinical-audit-research-and-service-review.pdf (accessed November 2022).

Broom, A. and Willis, E. (2007) Competing paradigms in health research, in M. Saks and J. Allsop (eds), *Researching Health: Qualitative, Quantitative and Mixed Methods*. London: Sage.

Bullivant, J. and Corbett-Nolan, A. (2010) Clinical audit: A simple guide for NHS boards and partners. London: Good Governance Institute.

Bullivant, J., Godfrey, K., Thorne, D., et al. (2015) *Clinical Audit: A Guide for NHS Boards and Partners*. London: Healthcare Quality Improvement Partnership and Good Governance Institute.

Centre for Reviews and Dissemination (CRD) (2009) Systematic reviews: CRD's guidance for undertaking reviews in health care. York: CRD. Available at: www.york.ac.uk/inst/crd/pdf/Systematic_Reviews.pdf (accessed January 2022).

Cochrane (n.d) About us. London: Cochrane. Available at: www.cochrane.org/about-us (accessed August 2023).

College of Operating Department Practitioners (CODP) (2006) Diploma in Higher Education in Operating Department Practice curriculum document. London: CODP.

College of Operating Department Practitioners (CODP) (2011) Bachelor of Science (Hons) in Operating Department Practice – England, Northern Ireland and Wales; Bachelor of Science in Operating Department Practice – Scotland. London: CODP.

College of Operating Department Practitioners (CODP) (2018) Bachelor of Science (Hons) in Operating Department Practice – England, Northern Ireland and Wales; Bachelor of Science in Operating Department Practice – Scotland: Curriculum document. London: CODP.

Copeland, G. (2005) A practical handbook for clinical audit: Guidance. London: Clinical Governance Support Team, NHS. Available at: https://citeseerx.ist.psu.edu/viewdoc/download?-doi=10.1.1.464.7819&rep=rep1&type=pdf (accessed January 2022).

Courtney, M., Rickard, C., Vickerstaff, J., et al. (2010) Evidence-based nursing practice, in M. Courney and H. McCutcheon (eds), *Using Evidence to Guide Nursing Practice*. Sydney: Churchill Livingstone.

Critical Appraisal Programme (CASP) (2021) CASP checklists. Oxford: CASP. Available at: www.casp-uk.net (accessed January 2022).

Cumpston, M., Flemyng, E., Thomas, J., et al. (2023) Introduction, in J.P.T. Higgins, J. Thomas, J. Chandler, et al. (eds), *Cochrane Handbook for Systematic Reviews of Interventions*, 2nd edn, Chapter 1. Chichester: John Wiley & Sons. Online *Handbook*, version 6.4 (updated August 2023). London: Cochrane. Available at: www.training.cochrane.org/handbook (accessed August 2023).

Department of Health (DH) (2009) Reference guide to consent for examination or treatment, 2nd edn. London: DH. Available at: https://assets.publishing.service.gov.uk/government/uploads/system/uploads/attachment_data/file/138296/dh_103653__1_.pdf (accessed January 2022).

Driessnack, M., Sousa, V.D. and Mendes, I.A.A. (2007) An overview of research designs relevant to nursing: Part 3: Mixed and multiple methods, *Revista Latino-Americana de enfermagem*, 15(5): 1046–9.

Gecaj-Gashi, A., Hashimi, M., Baftiu, N., et al. (2010) Propofol vs isoflurane anesthesia-incidence of PONV in patients at maxillofacial surgery, *Advances in Medical Science*, 55(2): 308–12.

Glaser, B.G. and Strauss, A.L. (1967) *Discovery of Grounded Theory: Strategies for Qualitative Research*. Chicago, IL: AldineTransaction.

Glasziou, P., Del Mar, C. and Salisbury, J. (2003) *Evidence-Based Medicine Workbook: Finding and Applying the Best Research Evidence to Improve Patient Care*. London: BMJ Books.

Grainger, A. (2010) Clinical audit: Shining a light on good practice, *Nursing Management*, 17(4): 30–3.

Health and Care Professions Council (HCPC) (2016) Standards of conduct, performance and ethics. London: HCPC.

Health and Care Professions Council (HCPC) (2023) Standards of proficiency: Operating Department Practitioners. London: HCPC.

Health Education England (HEE) (2022) Allied Health Professions' research and innovation strategy for England. Leicester: HEE. Available at: www.hee.nhs.uk/our-work/allied-health-professions/ enable-workforce/allied-health-professions%E2%80%99-research-innovation-strategy-england (accessed January 2022).

Healthcare Quality Improvement Partnership (HQIP) (2020) Best practice in clinical audit. London: HQIP.

Jones, K. (2007) Doing a literature review in health, in M. Saks and J. Allsop (eds), *Researching Health: Qualitative, Quantitative and Mixed Methods*. London: Sage.

Katz, M.H. (2006) *Study Design and Statistical Analysis: A Practical Guide for Clinicians*. Cambridge: Cambridge University Press.

King's Health Partners (2022) Audits and service evaluation. London: King's Health Partners Available at: www.kingshealthpartners.org/research/getstarted/audits-and-service-evaluation (accessed November 2022).

Länsimies-Antikainen, H., Laitinen, T., Rauramaa, R., et al. (2009) Evaluation of informed consent in health research: A questionnaire survey, *Scandinavian Journal of Caring Studies*, 24: 56–64.

Litva, A. and Jacoby, A. (2007) Qualitative research: Critical appraisal, in J.V. Craig and R.L. Smyth (eds), *The Evidence-Based Practice Manual for Nurses*, 2nd edn. Edinburgh: Churchill Livingstone.

LoBiondo-Wood, G. and Haber, J. (2006) *Nursing Research Methods and Critical Appraisal for Evidence Based Practice*. St Louis, MO: Mosby Elsevier.

Mendlinger, S. and Cwikel, J. (2008) Spiraling between qualitative and quantative data on women's health behaviours: A double helix model for mixed methods, *Qualitative Health Research*, 18(2): 280–93.

Morse, J. (2010) Simultaneous and sequential qualitative mixed method designs, *Qualitative Enquiry*, 16(6): 483–91.

Morse, J.M. and Niehaus, L. (2009) *Principles and Procedures of Mixed Methods Design*. Walnut Creek, CA: Left Coast Press.

National Institute for Health and Clinical Excellence (NICE) (2002) *Principles for Best Practice in Clinical Audit*. Oxford: Radcliffe Medical Press.

NHS and partners (n.d.) Evaluation Works Toolkit. Available at: https://nhsevaluationtoolkit.net/ evaluation-cycle (accessed November 2022).

NHS England (n.d.) Clinical audit. London: NHS England. Available at:https://nhsevaluationtoolkit.net/evaluation-cycle (accessed November 2022).

NHS Health Research Authority (NHS HRA) (2021a) UK policy framework for health and social care research. London: NHS HRA. Available at: www.hra.nhs.uk/planning-and-improving-research/policies-standards-legislation/uk-policy-framework-health-social-care-research/ uk-policy-framework-health-and-social-care-research (accessed January 2022).

NHS Health Research Authority (NHS HRA) (2021b) Research Ethics Service. London: NHS HRA. Available: at www.hra.nhs.uk/about-us/committees-and-services/res-and-recs (accessed January 2022).

NHS Health Research Authority (NHS HRA) (2022) Defining research table. London: NHS HRA. Available at: www.hra-decisiontools.org.uk/research/docs/DefiningResearchTable_Oct2022. pdf (accessed November 2022).

Östlund, U., Kidd, L., Wengström, Y., et al. (2011) Combining qualitative and quantitative research within mixed method research design: A methodological review, *International Journal of Nursing Studies*, 48: 369–83.

Parahoo, K. (2014) *Nursing Research: Principles, Process and Issues*, 3rd edn. Basingstoke: Palgrave Macmillan.

Patel, S. (2010) Achieving quality assurance through clinical audit, *Nursing Management*, 17(3): 28–35.

Prasun, M.A. (2013) Evidence-based practice, *Heart and Lung*, 42: 84.

PRISMA (2021) PRISMA transparent reporting of systematic reviews and meta-analysis. Available at: www.prisma-statement.org (accessed November 2022).

Sackett, D.L., Straus, S.E., Richardson, W.S., et al. (2001) *Evidence-Based Medicine: How to Practice and Teach EBM*. London: Churchill Livingstone.

Smith, L. and Dixon, L. (2009) Systematic reviews, in J. Neale (ed.), *Research Methods for Health and Social Care*. Basingstoke: Palgrave Macmillan.

Strange, F. (2001) The persistence of ritual in nursing practice, *Clinical Effectiveness in Nursing*, 5(4): 177–83.

Tritter, J. (2007) Mixed methods and multidisciplinary research in health care, in M. Saks and J. Allsop (eds), *Researching Health: Qualitative, Quantitative and Mixed Methods*. London: Sage.

Useful resources

Cochrane Training: https://training.cochrane.org
Council for Allied Health Professions Research (CAHPR): https://cahpr.csp.org.uk

3 Professional practice for Operating Department Practitioners

Stephen Wordsworth

Key topics

- What is meant by the term 'professional practice' and is the ODP role a profession?
- Professional values, judgement, decision-making and clinical reasoning as key qualities of professionals
- Professional practice related to medicines

- Legal, professional and regulatory accountability and the role of the Health Care and Professions Council (HCPC) in maintaining and supporting clinical conduct and competence
- The scope of practice and developing advanced practice

Introduction

This chapter outlines the concepts and meaning of 'professional practice' from different perspectives that are relevant to your practice. Included are different definitions of the term 'professional', what it means to undertake professional practice in healthcare settings and who we might expect to be included in this group. Starting with both historical and theoretical perspectives, current research and practice development are drawn on to address some contemporary and emerging themes that relate to the Operating Department Practitioner (ODP) role.

Also explored are themes such as the principles of professionalism, including legal and regulatory accountability in the context of statutory regulations and registration, and in the role and function of the Health and Care Professions Council (HCPC). The chapter concludes by considering key interrelated concepts, such as autonomy, delegation and supervision, in relation to advanced practice and fitness to practise from a regulatory perspective.

Why is this relevant?

Most ODPs would probably consider themselves to be professional and describe themselves as such in conversations or debates with other healthcare colleagues.

As a result of the COVID-19 pandemic and the broader application of the ODP skillset, there is now a much wider appreciation of the role, both inside and outside the perioperative setting, and our claim that we belong to a profession. This is certainly the case in universities, where the principles of professionalism (how we act and think) are embedded in the pre-registration curriculum and, hence, students develop this aspect during their studies. Most ODPs might even use the terms 'profession' and 'professional' to describe and explain what their job entails to family and friends, which is harder than it might first seem! Is the term 'professional' now rightly applied to ODPs or is it still used to justify or defend the role rather than as a positive statement about the difference we make to patient care?

One way to explore this question further is to consider and compare which other groups have gained professional status and why. This might seem obvious but, in fact, the terms 'profession' and 'professional' are contested as they are open to interpretation and therefore disagreement. The danger lies in suggesting that you belong to a profession purely because of symbolic importance or occupational rivalry rather than displaying the qualities that can have a positive impact on behaviour and practice.

The ODP role has been a statutory one, regulated by the HCPC since 2004, but has this changed the way we think and practise? It is easy to see how regulation and registration might be confused with issues of status, getting paid more, promotion or career development opportunities, rather than improvements in the care of our patients. That ODPs came under the remit of the chief Allied Health Professions in England in 2017 is recognition that in the National Health Service (NHS) in England, ODPs have an equal and important role to play as one of the 14 separate but complementary Allied Health Professions (AHPs).

While in some respects ODPs may not always practice with the same level of autonomy afforded to others, it is important to remember that with increased status comes greater responsibility, both individually and as a profession, along with a significant degree of accountability for both our actions and our omissions.

Stop and think

What qualities do you associate with being a professional? How might these relate to registration and the HCPC?

What is a 'profession'?

Before taking a more in-depth look at the implications of the impact of belonging to a profession and acting professionally on practice, there are some viewpoints that might help to broaden our understanding. From a sociological perspective, Friedson (1994: 13) tells us that, historically, professions have been seen as 'honoured servants of public need . . . distinguished by their orientation to serving the needs of the public through the schooled application of their unusual esoteric knowledge and complex skill'.

In the context of the NHS and healthcare, being part of a public service and serving the public's needs still seem relevant and are likely to resonate with most ODPs. So is the idea of 'schooling' – in other words, applying learning to skills and practices via higher education (HE). If no longer 'esoteric', then at least we should consider ODPs as having specialist and specific knowledge. While the language is outdated, so too is the context, as no longer is it the case that belonging to a profession is only extended to small number of people, who by default had the potential to restrict other occupational groups.

The global expansion of higher education (HE) and the relationship with highly skilled economies have played significant parts in the growth of new occupational groups, particularly in healthcare. For ODPs, this trajectory gathered pace with the development of the College of Operating Department Practitioners (CODP, formerly the Association of Operating Department Practitioners or AODP) and the initial HE curriculum in 2001. This was an attempt to codify a specific 'body of knowledge', elements of which may not always be exclusive to the work of ODPs, but which are at least shared by all ODPs.

Building on the ideas of why status and qualifications are important to the development of professions, sociologist Pierre Bourdieu argues that maintaining a profession's status is only possible because of what he describes as 'capital', which can be both gained and lost in the eyes of society. For Bourdieu (1984), 'capital' is a complex interplay of cultural and social advantages that develop over a period of time. Bourdieu (2006) also suggests that 'capital begets capital'. When you practice your profession, you need to make the most of the benefits that are afforded to you by capitalizing on social advantage and educational opportunities. This means access to networks of people and institutions who lead and shape services, as well as those who develop policies and strategy. Being on the inside comes with opportunities to develop and advance skills, knowledge and qualifications that would not ordinarily exist. Becoming a professional allows you to accumulate more capital by benefiting from being involved, which, in turn, brings additional benefits and opportunities, and so your professional capital increases further. Over time, this interplay of advantage and opportunity leads to recognition, acceptance, status and even esteem.

Theorizing the professions

Bourdieu predicts that some professions (or social groups) are able to impose their status more than others. In other words, they use the capital that they have gained more effectively than others. We see this in the hierarchies that can exist in operating theatres. The theory of capital can also be useful as a way to explore the historical differences in status between ODPs and perioperative nurses and how occupational tensions can remain while ODPs, as a profession, are still engaged in gaining capital.

The idea of capital is perhaps better known through the work of Karl Marx. In his view, capital is based on the relative value of skills and knowledge to economic production and the wealth of a nation (Macdonald 1995). Marx might suggest that the true value of ODPs lies not in their contribution to patient care but to the wider healthcare economy and to the preservation of the government's ability to maintain the NHS.

Theorizing about the professions also materializes in the work of Foucault (1977). In his words, there is a 'genealogy' between the power of the state and legal systems to hold others to account. Indeed, the relationship between the work of government and the courts is necessary to uphold the needs of the public and society as a whole. In exchange for becoming part of the established order, some occupations receive a form of state patronage or privilege. This same process, in Foucauldian terms, is what underpins statutory regulations and the existence of the General Medical Council (GMC), HCPC and Nursing and Midwifery Council (NMC) to hold their registrants to account. Although independent from the government, they would not exist if it were not for the legal powers that the government grants them.

Ultimately, it is this same process that led to the regulation of ODPs. Our particular genealogy as a profession moved forwards in 2000, when the then NHS Executive issued guidance that handed legitimacy to the CODP to ensure that all ODPs working in the NHS submitted to a voluntary scheme of registration, which, a little while later, became statutory.

Critics of this process, while not necessarily objecting to individual professions, have argued that the state now dictates professional status on its own terms. Many of the advantages that accrued historically to professions which developed over time are not available to groups that become professions under this form of state endorsement. Timmons (2011) argues that, in reality, the endorsement of new health professions is limited only to regulation. Gone are the privileges associated with power, status and public esteem, which have been replaced by a system of accountability that is restrictive, intrusive and even anti-democratic.

In a report undertaken by the HCPC (2011: 4), it, too, recognizes the changing context of what it means to be a professional (which it refers to throughout the report as professionalism) and, at the same time, the HCPC sets the tone for its future approach to regulation. The HCPC acknowledges that the newly 'professionalized' may find it harder to gain the kind of support and recognition that long-established professions enjoy, and this is often contingent on the specific nature and context. The concept of a more contemporary view of professionalism is a dynamic judgement rather than a discrete and static skill set. Looking at professional attributes in this way opens up the possibility of exploring models of professionalism that move away from elitist, hierarchical and, more often than not, patriarchal positions (Witz 1992).

New debates around professionalism

So far, we have seen how traditional definitions provide a rather fixed construction of the notion of what a profession is. A number of commentators have suggested that this is still the case in the medical profession, where a focus on expert knowledge remains paramount (Cruess and Cruess 2006; Stern 2006). Furthermore, such static definitions ignore the fact that the spotlight is now not only on the skills and knowledge of members of the profession but on their attitudes, values and behaviours. In short, on their *professionalism* as a whole. The study on professionalism carried out by the HCPC (2011) remains an important milestone in identifying several key dimensions that help to frame a more contemporary discussion of professionalism and professional practice. The study is also significant because it captures not only registrant views from 12 different professions but also the views of future practitioners (students) and managers alike.

Stop and think

What kinds of qualities come to mind when you think about your role as a professional? Can you list some characteristics and personal attributes that are needed to provide effective and compassionate patient care?

Professionalism is best expressed as a whole, as an all-encompassing concept, rather than a discrete set of unrelated characteristics. It can be likened to an overall way of being that comprises a range of skills, attitudes and behaviours. In the HCPC (2011) study, this concept also came across in the way that participants considered their role reflexively, commenting not on their individual attributes but on how they would like to be treated if they were the patient or service user. In a separate study looking into career choices, students articulated this same desire, to care for patients according to how they would like to be cared for themselves. These students were motivated by the desire to help others who need the care and support of a professional. Indeed, these students were motivated to join their chosen profession by the desire to be able to 'improve the quality of people's lives' as a holistic view of the role rather than simply to cure a particular problem (Wordsworth 2015).

Professionalism as good clinical care

Despite a greater emphasis today on behaviours, the need to demonstrate technical skills and competence is still important to the way in which professionals and professionalism are viewed. Again, findings from the HCPC (2011) study stressed the importance of an ongoing 'ability to do the job'. However, the pace at which roles are changing, often driven by technological developments, means that keeping up with new competencies can be problematic. Therefore, in many ways, the essence of practice is concerned with the ability of practitioners to know and understand their limitations, so they can seek out ways to keep their skills up to date and recognize when this is not the case. Again, in the parallel study on student choice (Wordsworth, 2015), a number of participants felt that they would be more useful, trusted and 'part of the team' the more technically competent they became. Their peers judged them on their apparent skills and not on their behaviours and attitudes. This is also evident when ODPs seek to extend their scope of practice or move to advanced practice roles, where they are expected to learn and perform new and enhanced technical skills, as well as develop new knowledge and the application of this to complex activities. Developing practice, for example, is reduced to learning new skills in isolation from autonomous thinking to enable greater patient advocacy.

No wonder the perioperative environment can often feel very intense. The constant drive for high degrees of technical and clinical competence can lead to stressful situations and lack of compassion.

Professional values

Given the types of professional attributes and behaviours that can be seen, the HCPC study (2011: 12) reported that this was related to the context in which the professional was practising and where this was taking place, in the NHS, for example, or in the independent healthcare sector. The study also identified that the variability was shaped by the individuals themselves, as they demonstrated different personal qualities and values, creating 'a dynamic tension for developing and judgement of professionalism, which comes down to personal and internalised beliefs . . . situated in the immediate environment'.

On occasions, through fitness to practise cases, it is evident that there are times when an individual's values and behaviours fall short of the standard required. In extreme circumstances, we can even see when institutional and systems failures enable unacceptable professional values and behaviours to become normalized, as was the case at the Mid Staffordshire NHS Foundation Trust. The Francis inquiry (Francis 2013) found that the organization condoned unacceptable behaviours, including lack of empathy, bullying, a culture of secrecy and a lack of candour (openness and honesty), as well as denial in refusing to accept that anything was wrong and improvement was needed.

The lack of professional characteristics displayed by some staff also extended to poor communication and attitudes towards patients, their families and visitors, which were essential for all those most in need of care and compassion from the Trust. These are the very antithesis of Wilkinson et al.'s (2009) positive professional attributes, cited as:

- adherence to ethical practice;
- effective interactions with patients and service users;
- effective interactions with staff;
- reliability and commitment to improvement.

The findings of the Francis inquiry (2013) led to the development of a vision and set of values known as the '6 Cs', which are care, compassion, competence, communication, courage, and commitment (DH and NHS Commissioning Board 2012).

The 6 Cs affirm what can be considered to be a set of personal qualities that each individual brings to their expression of professionalism. Words such as caring, compassion, empathy, respect and dignity are used to describe what is expected of the professional putting these qualities into action. How they are then embedded in professional practice depends on a number of factors, including educational and social encounters, past experiences, plus cultural and familial backgrounds.

Professional judgement and decision-making

Professional values often shape our moral and ethical viewpoints and, therefore, how, as ODPs, we arrive at patient-centred decision-making. What might be considered value judgements stem in part from social and cultural norms, such as our beliefs, religious practices and upbringing. ODPs might find that some of the clinical decisions they are involved with, while legally acceptable, may not fit with their own moral or ethical viewpoint. Indeed, there may be times when ODPs are asked to participate in a particular episode of care that they are not comfortable with or may even have objections to. However, as a professional, you may be asked to reach an informed and reasonable decision based on the interests of the patient.

Moral and ethical dilemmas

When undertaking clinical decision-making in situations where there is ambiguity around what is in the best interests of the patient, Griffith and Tengnah (2010) argue that it is essential such professional dilemmas are understood so they can inform professional practice, particularly where those dilemmas may conflict with their personal values. For example, an ODP might have a moral objection to certain surgical procedures (such as the termination of pregnancy when they believe in the sanctity of life) or they may not agree with a patient's decision and legal right to refuse further surgery.

In such circumstances, it can be beneficial to apply ethical principles to the moral dilemma. Beauchamp and Childress's (1989) is perhaps the most accessible and widely applicable model to guide a professional decision and course of action. The stages, or principles, included in the model are respect for autonomy (make their own choice), non-maleficence (in best interests of others), beneficence (do no harm) and justice (fairness and equality).

Stop and think

Do you have the courage and commitment to speak up to improve the patient's experience? How would you go about raising your concerns surrounding poor care?

Clinical reasoning as a professional competence

The skill of ODPs in being able to relate and communicate effectively can undoubtedly reduce patients' anxiety, which, in turn, can have a positive impact on their psychological and physical responses. Atkins and Ersser (2008) argue that clinical reasoning skills and effective communication are necessary for good ethical care but can also directly influence clinical effectiveness and outcomes.

The various models of professional practice convey differences in the degree of importance placed on the relationship between patients and professionals. The perioperative environment raises specific challenges to the notion of patient involvement and participation in their own care and treatment. As an alternative, Charles et al. (1999) advocate a shared decision-making approach, in which the role of the healthcare professional is to guide and support the patient to reach the decision that is right for them. By contrast, enabling 'informed choice' stresses both the positive benefits and risks of treatment as being the key responsibility of the healthcare professional, and in the perioperative environment this usually remains the responsibility of the medical team. If this were to change, the development of clinical reasoning may require the ODP to act more as a conduit and resource for information, to complement their technical skills. Greater involvement in clinical reasoning as a key professional responsibility would be to help educate and inform patients to enable them to get involved in their treatment (Entwistle 2000). In short, ODPs, as part of the development of their profession, should recognize their potential contribution to furthering the long-term health and well-being of their patients.

Professionalism as an expression of self

Another finding of the HCPC (2011) study was that the notion of professionalism is somehow intrinsically linked to the expression of self. In the minds of practitioners and educators alike, 'being a professional' was a deeply held 'core belief' that defined their actions and thoughts, a quality that underpinned their practice through their own pre-existing meta-qualities. Importantly, the (HCPC 2011: 15) study demonstrates how being a professional is often viewed as being 'a way of life'. In this context, it is not possible to stop being a professional at the point that practitioners finish their shift. In fact, participants from a range of professions regulated by the HCPC felt strongly that key professional qualities and behaviours extend to all aspects of their lives, both at and outside of work. Inevitably, this could lead to a lack of clarity as to how far one's personal life should be influenced by the need to act and behave professionally at all times. Respondents taking part in the HCPC (2011: 15) study were aware of a blurring between the 'professional and private self'. This has important consequences in relation to the conduct of ODPs, as well as the role of the regulator in holding a practitioner to account for their lack of professionalism. Over time, this has led to the idea that being a professional is less about qualifications and competence, and more about a practitioner's values and behaviours.

The best way to demonstrate where the professional and personal can become blurred is in the case of social media, as in this area the most contemporary questions can come up regarding what it means to be a professional. It is worth noting that engaging with social media can bring many benefits, such as professionals, including ODPs, taking to social media to like, comment and follow, as well as blog or post videos, about their role. Many actively engage in conversations with employers and members of the public about what their skills enable them to do. Not only can social media platforms be used to raise the profile of the profession but they can also be a useful tool in networking with others, disseminating professional knowledge and even as a platform for research and innovation. However, when used inappropriately, social media is a significant factor in an increasing number of fitness to practise concerns and allegations, as well as investigations into the conduct of employees by employers.

Stop and think

Can you think of any situations both at and outside work involving social media that might have a negative impact on your professionalism and practice? What kind of activities and actions should you avoid?

The HCPC has produced guidance for registrants plus some tips, listed below, and these are a useful starting point for considering best practice regarding the use of social media and how to avoid unprofessional use. Navigating on the HCPC's website to the section 'Meeting our standards' (2021c), there is a further section on 'Guidance on the use of social media' (2020a).

- **Think before you post.** Take a moment – the second you post, it can be seen by everyone.
- **Think about who can see what you share.** Take a moment to actively manage your privacy settings, otherwise you cannot guarantee that what you post won't be available to everyone.
- **Maintain appropriate professional boundaries.** Take a moment to consider that you could be communicating with not only colleagues but also patients, parents and family members alike.
- **Do not post information that is confidential or identifies patients.** Take a moment to consider whether you should share information if it may be confidential or sensitive.
- **Do not post inappropriate or offensive material.** Take a moment to use your professional judgment and ask whether what you share is in keeping with the standards that are expected of you as a professional.
- **Do not post anything that is likely to breach your contract of employment.** Take a moment to ensure that what you share is permissible and follows your employer's policies.
- **If in doubt, don't post or share.** Take a moment to seek advice. This could be from a colleague or perhaps a trade union or a professional body, such as the HCPC or CODP.

Inappropriate use of social media can raise concerns about your integrity as a professional and that you are bringing your profession and your employer into disrepute. This makes it important that you are aware of not only the benefits but also the pitfalls of social media, particularly in the context of how its use relates the standards set out by the HCPC (see Table 3.1).

The HCPC's 'Standards of conduct, performance and ethics' (2016a) are generic standards that apply to each of the professions the HCPC regulates. The standards are designed to express what is expected of each registrant in terms of how they present themselves publicly and professionally. These particular standards define the regulatory basis on which ODPs' values, behaviour and character should be based. They codify many of the attributes that were previously identified in the HCPC (2011) study on professionalism. They should also act as a guide for ODPs as to how to make the right decisions about their conduct and care of their patients.

One further area of performance and conduct that intersects with practitioners' values and behaviours is the increased attention that has been drawn by the HCPC to questions of equality, diversity and inclusion (EDI). The development of a specific strategy set out by the HCPC (2021b) is intent on eliminating harassment and victimization and ensuring the equality of opportunity for registrants, service users, colleagues and partners. In committing to ensure that their regulatory decisions and processes are free from bias and discrimination, ODPs should

Table 3.1 How to use social media and adhere to the HCPC's 'Standards of conduct, performance and ethics' (2016a)

Standard	Key issue	Consideration
5.1 You must treat information about a service user as confidential	Confidentiality	Confidentiality is central to your professional practice. Should you be sharing personal information on social media? If it is about a patient, do you have their consent?
2.7 You must use all forms of communication appropriately and responsibly, including social media and networking websites	Communication	Are you able to apply the same standard to social media as you would in other forms of communication? You should be polite and respectful. Avoid inappropriate or offensive language
9.1 You must make sure that your conduct justifies the public's trust and confidence in you and your profession	Honesty and trustworthiness	Be careful about what you share. Even if you intend it to be personal, what you share may be seen by your employer, colleagues and patients
9.3 You must make sure that any promotional activities you are involved in are accurate and not likely to mislead	Honesty and trustworthiness	If you choose to share any information, make sure it is accurate and not misleading. Tell the truth and be clear that they are your views and not those of your employer
1.7 You must keep your relationships with service users and carers professional	Appropriate boundaries	Be mindful not to blur boundaries between your personal and professional life. Communicate in a professional manner. If you plan to engage directly with patients, you should first agree whether this is appropriate with your employer
		It may be more appropriate to decline or reject follows, as patients may still be able to find and contact you via your personal account. Consider letting them know that you cannot mix social and professional relationships. If you wish to follow up any contact you receive, consider using a more secure communication channel
		Social media and networking platforms are evolving rapidly and as use of these tools increases, this can lead to the blurring of lines between professional and personal use

feel able to speak out about discrimination in all of its forms, and ask questions and 'challenge in a way that encourages constructive conversation and supports positive change' (HCPC 2020b). Where issues related to EDI contribute to discrimination or lack of fairness, either consciously or unconsciously, then not only is the conduct and performance of individuals to be called into question but this also reflects negatively on the profession as a whole.

Together, the Standards of conduct, performance and ethics, along with the Standards of education and training, Standards of continuing professional development and Standards of proficiency, form a basis for the HCPC to act and carry out its function as a statutory regulator. In effect, these standards set out the foundations of what is expected of you legally, ethically and professionally as a registered ODP.

The HCPC and the ODP

Expressing what is expected of you in the form of standards is principally a form of accountability. Accountability in healthcare is there primarily to ensure the public is protected from acts or omissions that might cause harm (Wordsworth 2007). ODPs can be called to account if their conduct and, indeed, competence falls below expected standards.

Alongside accountability to your employer and the law, ODPs are also accountable to what is termed a 'higher authority' – in this case, it is the HCPC (Wordsworth 2014). The HCPC came into being as a result of the provisions of the Health and Social Work Order 2001, which itself was made under section 60 of the Health Act 1999. The order was also subject to further revocations and amendments in 2003. However, the inclusion of the role of ODP as a statutory regulated profession was the result of additional legislation in the form of the Health Professions (Operating Department Practitioners and Miscellaneous Amendments) Order 2004.

The HCPC is an independent regulator (separate from the government) of multiple professions and its purpose is to protect the public. In broad terms, it does this through setting standards; it approves the education programmes that must be completed before an individual can register with the HCPC and it keeps a register of professionals, taking action when anyone on the register does not meet its standards, primarily via the fitness to practise process.

While most of the standards (see Figure 3.1) apply directly to ODPs, the 'Standards of education and training' (HCPC 2017) specifically address what is expected from HE establishments that offer education and training programmes approved by the HCPC. As a student, learner or apprentice, these standards set out what you can expect from your education provider and from the programme that you are studying. Perhaps the most significant development regarding these standards for ODPs has been the consultation and subsequent change to the threshold qualification, which is now set at degree level (HCPC 2021a).

Alongside the 'Standards of conduct, performance and ethics' (HCPC 2016a), which, as we have seen, provide a basis for professional practice, the 'Standards of continuing professional development' (HCPC 2018a) provide a mechanism by which registrants can maintain, update and record their professional development throughout their careers, as well as demonstrate how this benefits patients. If asked, registrants should also be ready to submit to an audit of their continuing professional development (CPD).

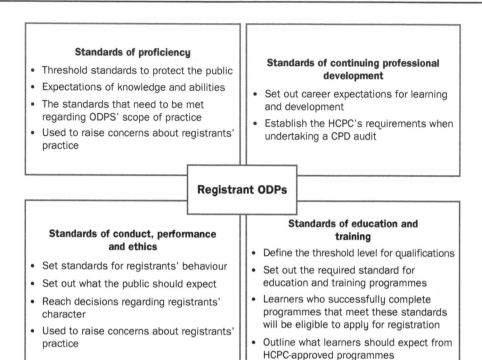

Standards of proficiency

- Threshold standards to protect the public
- Expectations of knowledge and abilities
- The standards that need to be met regarding ODPS' scope of practice
- Used to raise concerns about registrants' practice

Standards of continuing professional development

- Set out career expectations for learning and development
- Establish the HCPC's requirements when undertaking a CPD audit

Registrant ODPs

Standards of conduct, performance and ethics

- Set standards for registrants' behaviour
- Set out what the public should expect
- Reach decisions regarding registrants' character
- Used to raise concerns about registrants' practice

Standards of education and training

- Define the threshold level for qualifications
- Set out the required standard for education and training programmes
- Learners who successfully complete programmes that meet these standards will be eligible to apply for registration
- Outline what learners should expect from HCPC-approved programmes

Figure 3.1.

Stop and think

What kinds of activity are you involved in that could count as CPD if you were asked to submit to an audit of this? How could this develop you as a professional?

While these standards relate to registrants, students on approved education and training programmes must also consider how their ethical practice and professional development enables them to achieve their professional standards The HCPC (2016b) has produced 'Guidance on conduct and ethics for students'. This mirrors its 'Standards of conduct, performance and ethics' (HCPC 2016a) The HCPC (2022), via its student hub, has produced additional guidance on CPD for students following either formal or self-directed means of keeping up to date via work-based and professional activities.

Perhaps the standards that most ODPs, and, indeed, all registrants, are more familiar with are the 'Standards of proficiency' (SoPs; HCPC 2023). Those for operating department practice are threshold standards, to be achieved at the point of registration. Students who have completed a recognized training programme should be aware that they are not registered automatically, but are eligible to apply to be entered on to the register (subject to meeting the conditions of good health and character). Once registered, ODPs must be able to demonstrate, at the point of each registration renewal cycle of two years, that they have met the requirements of their CPD standards within the scope of their practice.

Stop and think

Have you ever been concerned by something that you have been asked to do or by working practices? Have you ever questioned the currency of your own knowledge or practice? Consider how this might affect your registration and what action you would take in the future.

Again, the link between what are now considered to be core professional and personal attributes and the need to keep knowledge and skills up to date are clearly prescribed as 'must dos' in standards, as is recognizing that maintaining your own health is paramount to safe and effective care. To enable you to decide how you meet the standards, the HCPC (2021c) advises that:

> As an autonomous professional, you need to make informed, reasoned decisions about your practice to ensure that you meet the standards that apply to you. This includes seeking advice and support from education providers, employers, colleagues, professional bodies, unions and others to ensure that the wellbeing of service users is safeguarded at all times. So long as you do this and can justify your decisions if asked to, it is very unlikely that you will not meet our standards.

Where this is found not to be the case, the HCPC has the ability to hold registered professionals to account via its 'fitness to practise' process (HCPC 2018b). In broad terms, if there are concerns over a registrant's fitness to practise, a preliminary investigation can be undertaken to assess whether 'there is a case to answer'. If there is, the matter will be referred to a hearing, which will take place in one of the following committees:

- a conduct and competence committee for cases concerning misconduct, lack of competence convictions or cautions, decisions by other regulators and barring decisions;
- a panel of the health committee for cases where the health of the ODP may be affecting their ability to practise.

In cases where there is evidence that a registrant's fitness to practise is impaired, the Health Professions Order (2001) 29(c) makes provisions that enable either of these committees to:

- make an order directing the registrar to strike the person concerned off the register (a 'striking-off order');
- make an order directing the registrar to suspend the registration of the person for a specified period, not exceeding a year (a 'suspension order');
- make an order imposing conditions the person must comply with for a specified period, not exceeding three years (a 'conditions of practice order');
- caution the person and make an order directing the registrar to annotate the register accordingly for a specified period, not less than a year and not more than five years (a 'caution order').

That you continue to meet the standards and how this can be maintained is often associated with your 'scope of practice'. This may well be different for each ODP, according to their role, experience and the institution they work in.

The scope of practice for ODPs

Given the professional context of the perioperative environment, including changes to medical staffing and training of junior doctors, advances in technology and patient demographics, it is reasonable to assume that the role of the ODP will continue to develop over time. The scope of practice has been extended to roles in the operating theatre as well as outside the historical boundaries of perioperative care and, typically, can include the following roles:

- surgical care practitioner;
- surgical pre-assessment practitioner;
- resuscitation officer;
- transplant co-ordinator;
- specialist ophthalmic anaesthetic practitioner.

Many ODPs also extend their scope of practice themselves, in the sense that they specialize in either educational or leadership roles in the NHS and independent healthcare sector, as well as in HE. Many ODPs are now increasingly involved in research, clinical audits and service improvement. During the COVID-19 pandemic, many ODPs were redeployed by the NHS to critical care areas, where they were able to use their airway management and care of the ventilated patient training and skills. Although ODPS have worked in critical care areas for some time, the pandemic raised the profile of the profession and demonstrated the possibilities for the extension of the scope of practice into other clinical areas.

Anticipating the inevitable development of the current 'Scope of practice' (CODP 2009), the CODP (2010: 5) has considered how ODPs can remain occupationally competent:

> As the healthcare environment continues to change, practitioners [ODPs] are required to maintain and develop their competence, to develop their knowledge base as knowledge changes and expands, and to adapt their skills to new circumstances in which they find themselves.

In developing your own scope of practice, it is paramount that you undertake the following self-assessment to comply with the legal, ethical and regulatory mechanisms of accountability.

- Do I consider that I am participating in a reasonable and justifiable course of treatment or intervention?
- Am I aware of, and have considered, any evidenced-based practice?
- To participate competently in the care of the patient, do I have the necessary knowledge, skills and experience?
- Am I able to demonstrate professional development and fitness to practise by maintaining my CPD?

In summary, the scope of practice can be seen as defining the limits of your current knowledge, skills and experience. It will therefore depend on how much appropriate education and training you have received and how much you will need to do to extend your current role. Your scope of practice may be restricted by law – is it legal for you to do what you would like to do? This last aspect will arise particularly with regard to prescribing. Finally, to extend your scope of practice, you should ensure that you have appropriate professional indemnity cover for the activity you wish to undertake.

The dynamic nature of the scope of practice is best exemplified by developments in more recent years that have resulted in the role evolving in the operating theatre but also in roles outside the perioperative environment. In the UK's response to the COVID-19 pandemic, for example, the ODPs' skill set was used in a number of clinical settings outside operating theatres.

Advanced practice and ODPs

An increasing number of healthcare professions, including ODPs as we have seen, are undertaking new or additional roles beyond their traditional scope of practice. Typically, these roles can be shared with other professionals, including doctors, nurses and other AHPs, with whom elements of the body of knowledge can also be shared as a result of their clinical roles.

In the UK, advanced clinical practitioners (ACPs) are usually employed in the NHS and independent healthcare sectors. ACP roles began to increase following the Nuffield Trust report, 'Reshaping the workforce to deliver the care patients need' (Imison 2016), the aim of which was to provide guidance on the development of the non-medical workforce to ensure service provision needs could be met at a time of increasing demand. Although, in truth, that was already being talked about sometime earlier, as a result of changes to junior doctors' contracts, including working hours and the move away from the traditional educational models (McGee 2009).

There is agreement from a policy perspective across all four nations of the UK on the four pillars of advanced practice as a means of transforming and modernizing 'pathways of care', enabling the safe and effective sharing of skills across traditional professional boundaries (HEE 2017). The four pillars of advanced practice are:

- expert clinical practice
- leadership and management
- education and training
- research, audit and service evaluation.

However, in practice, as roles have developed, some pillars have been afforded more emphasis than others, depending on the needs of organizations, roles and clinical need, as well as job titles and descriptions. While most commentators agree that some consistency is evident, in terms of leadership, education and research, this is less so when describing the elements of the role that are specifically to do with the advanced level of practice (East et al. 2015).

Presenting the nursing model of advanced practice has come to dominate the debate, which is understandable given the scale of the nursing workforce and sheer variety of roles they fulfil. This model of development has no doubt been helped by the fact that advance practice in nursing has emerged through a single professional lens, unlike those for the AHP workforce, in which each profession may have a different perspective and its professional body's perspective may be different again. Despite the development of non-medical advanced practice, it is fair to say that the evidence to support better patient outcomes is still emerging (Saxon et al. 2014). What is not in dispute is the fact that there is a growing level of recognition of the role and its importance in meeting workforce needs and its potential for enhanced patient care.

In the case of AHP advanced practice, in a research study carried out on behalf of the HCPC, Hardy (2021) found that, of the HCPC-regulated professions, there was a lack of consistency and definition of the scope of advanced practice. The same was true of role titles, with different titles being used, inconsistently, and variations in the underpinning educational qualifications and experience required for entry to these roles or in support of the development of advanced knowledge and skills. Based on the report, the HCPC (2021a) concluded that there was not yet a compelling case for separate statutory regulations or any specific need for additional forms of protection of the public, such as annotation of the register. This is likely to change in time, but will require some degree of agreement and collaboration between AHPs to make further safe and effective regulation possible.

Given the context of operating theatres and the demands for more operating time, the advances in technology and surgical and anaesthetic services, alongside changes to junior doctors' roles, it is clear that advanced practice should have an important role to play in future designs for the workforce and mix of skills to meet demand. In many ways, of all those working in perioperative and surgical care, ODPs are perhaps best equipped to carry out advanced practice roles. The extent to which this is taking place is evident in Hardy's (2021) research study. A total of 285 ODPs participated in the study and, of those, 69 indicated that they were working at or training for some form of advance practice. Many of the respondents indicated that increasing numbers of ODPs are practising beyond the perioperative environment in a variety of settings, including wards and clinics. More than half the respondents also indicated that they were in leadership roles to complement those of advanced practice. Although not an exhaustive list, ODPs typically cited the following pre-pandemic developments in roles:

- advanced critical care practitioner
- advanced clinical practitioner (clinics and wards)
- surgical assistant
- emergency department practitioner
- anaesthesia associate
- endoscopy practitioner.

With further recognition of the ODPs' skill set being extended to include the assessment and triage in trauma and resuscitation, pre-hospital, community roles encompassing solo responder, as well as offshore health professional roles, patient transfer and retrieval, including co-ordinator and live donor programme leadership responsibilities.

A growing number of ODPs are also working in aesthetic services, undertaking non-surgical cosmetic procedures. As this typically takes place in the independent healthcare sector, as a sole trader or business, it is vital that practitioners are indemnified for the range of treatments offered and the devices and equipment used. ODPs working in this area must continue to practise within the parameters of the HCPC's 'Standards of conduct, performance and ethics' (2016). Additionally, best practice and training guidelines, as well as the standards of practice of the Cosmetic Practice Standards Authority (CPSA) apply to anyone undertaking aesthetic treatments. A registration scheme approved by the Professional Standards Agency (PSA) is also operated by the Joint Council for Cosmetic Practitioners (JCCP).

The ODP professions and medicines

Under the current legislation, ODPs are able to use patient-specific directions (PSDs) to administer or supply a medicine. A PSD is a written instruction to administer a medicine to a named patient who has been assessed by the authorized prescriber, who then prescribes the medicine. As a PSD applies to each individual patient, it is easy to see how this might, in certain circumstances, be burdensome and lead to delays and have an impact on the quality of patient outcomes and care, as well as the patient experience.

In this case, the duty of care lies with the prescriber, who remains legally accountable for the care they provide and for any delegation. For an ODP to be able to administer prescription-only medicines (POMS) under a PSD, the prescriber must be satisfied that they have the qualifications, experience, knowledge and skills to provide the care or treatment required.

A patient group direction (PGD) is a form of written instruction for medicines, including some controlled drugs, to be supplied and/or administered by some health professionals to a specified group of patients without a prescription or PSD being necessary. ODPs need to be clear on the following and ensure that there is clarity about the implementation of PGDs at service level:

- ODPs should be actively involved in the writing and authorization of PGDs;
- assurance of competence to supply and/or administer the medicine(s) should be included in the PGD by the service lead;
- the local protocol should include an overarching view of PGDs used in the organization concerned;
- there needs to be compliance with audits of use and impact.

At the point that ODPs have been given and are able to use a PGD to enable them to carry out advanced roles and patient care, this still does not entitle them to be considered non-medical prescribers (NMP). There are three different types of NMPs: independent prescribing, supplementary prescribing and prescribing by community practitioner nurse prescribers according to the *Nurse Prescribers' Formulary* (Nurse Prescribers' Advisory Group 2018).

During the pandemic, a specific protocol was introduced to ensure that the UK had a workforce of a sufficient size to deliver a COVID-19 vaccination programme. This required specific regulation changes to be made to the Human Medicines

Regulations 2012 via the Human Medicines (Coronavirus and Influenza) (Amendment) Regulations 2020. Acting similarly to a PGD, this allows the supply or administration of a COVID-19 vaccine, and for it to be administered by trained and competent non-registered healthcare workers as well as registered healthcare professionals.

Many ODPs were at the forefront of the national response to the pandemic. Not only has this raised the profile of the profession more generally but it has also shone a light on the ODP skill set and the professional way in which ODPs are able to apply and adapt their knowledge and skills to wherever they are needed.

Conclusion

According to contemporary debates about professions and professionalism, ODPs have now rightly made a successful case for being considered to be a profession. This may bring individual benefits but it also comes with additional responsibilities and requirements. Key characteristics define what it is to belong to a profession and practise as a professional. These can be far reaching and extend to both professional and personal behaviours, values and attributes.

Professionalism, as both a concept and in practice, is closely linked to regulation and registration, and the awareness of and adherence to standards is paramount to ensuring that ODPs maintain the standards expected of them. In the context of contemporary healthcare, it is very likely that the ODPs' scope of practice will continue to develop. Events such as the pandemic have highlighted just how effectively the skills of ODPs can be utilized in new ways to meet patients' needs. Knowing when to develop or advance one's practice is itself a characteristic of a profession. There are many paths that this can take, but we must also be cognisant of our own accountability. Hurdles still remain but progress is being made. Perhaps this chapter will stimulate debates on these points and act as a catalyst for further investigation and research from other ODPs to contribute to this much needed aspect of the role.

Key points

- Professionalism should be viewed as a set of characteristics and qualities that transcend your professional status and any hierarchy.
- Demonstrating the right values and behaviours personally and professionally should be central to the practice of all ODPs.
- Accountability is an important consequence of professionalism that links to a number of professional and statutory standards of conduct.
- The scope of practice relates to both professional and individual practitioner's roles, which should naturally change and within an awareness of their scope of practice.
- Advanced practice has the potential to improve the care of the patient. ODPs should contribute to this within legal professional boundaries and guidelines.
- ODPs should understand how administration of medicines and prescribing can shape their practice now, and for the future.

References and further reading

Association of Operating Department Practitioners (AODP) (2001) Diploma (HE) in Operating Department Practice: Curriculum document. Lewes: AODP.

Atkins, S. and Ersser, J.S. (2008) Clinical reasoning and patient-centred care, in J. Higgs, M.A. Jones, S. Loftus et al. (eds), *Clinical Reasoning in the Health Professions*, 3rd edn. London: Elsevier, Butterworth, Heinemann.

Beauchamp, T. and Childress, J. (1989) *Principles of Biomedical Ethics*. Oxford: Oxford University Press.

Bourdieu, P. (1984) *Distinction: A Social Critique of the Judgement of Taste*. R. Nice (trans.). London: Routledge & Kegan Paul.

Bourdieu, P. (2006) The forms of capital, in H. Lauder, P. Brown, J.A. Dillaborough and A.H. Halsey (eds), *Education, Globalisation and Social Change*. Oxford: Oxford University Press.

Charles, C., Gafni, A. and Whelan, T. (1999) Decision-making in the physician–patient encounter: Revisiting the shared treatment decision-making model, *Social Sciences and Medicine*, 49: 651–61.

College of Operating Department Practitioners (CODP) (2009) Scope of practice. London: CODP.

College of Operating Department Practitioners (CODP) (2010) Discussion paper: Framing the future role and function of Operating Department Practitioners. London: CODP.

Cruess, R.L. and Cruess, S.R. (2006) Teaching professionalism: General principles, *Medical Teacher*, 28: 205–8.

Department of Health (DH) and NHS Commissioning Board (2012) Compassion in practice: Nursing, midwifery and care staff: Our vision and strategy. London: DH and NHS Commissioning Board. Available at: www.england.nhs.uk/wp-content/uploads/2012/12/compassion-in-practice.pdf (accessed November 2022).

East, L., Knowles, K., Pettman, M., et al. (2015) Advanced level nursing in England: Organisational challenges and opportunities, *Journal of Nursing Management*, 23: 1011–19.

Entwistle, V.A. (2000) Supporting and resourcing treatment decision-making: Some policy considerations, *Health Expectations*, 3: 77–85.

Foucault, M. (1977) *Discipline and Punishment: The Birth of the Prison*. London: Penguin.

Francis, R. (2013) Report of the Mid Staffordshire NHS Foundation Trust public inquiry: Executive summary. HC 947. London: The Stationery Office. Available at: https://assets.publishing.service.gov.uk/government/uploads/system/uploads/attachment_data/file/279124/0947.pdf (accessed September 2022).

Friedson, E. (1994) *Professions Reborn: Theory, Prophecy and Policy*. Cambridge: Polity Press.

Griffith, R. and Tengnah, C. (2010) *Law and Professional Issues in Nursing*, 2nd edn. Exeter: Learning Matters.

Hardy, M. (2021) Advanced practice: Research report. London: Health and Care Professions Council (HCPC). Available at: www.hcpc-uk.org/resources/policy/advanced-practice-full-research-report (accessed November 2022).

Health and Care Professions Council (HCPC) (2011) Professionalism in healthcare professionals: Research report. London: HCPC. Available at: www.hcpc-uk.org/resources/reports/2011/professionalism-in-healthcare-professionals (accessed November 2022).

Health and Care Professions Council (HCPC) (2016a) Standards of conduct, performance and ethics. London: HCPC. Available at: www.hcpc-uk.org/standards/standards-of-conduct-performance-and-ethics (accessed November 2022).

Health and Care Professions Council (HCPC) (2016b) Guidance on conduct and ethics for students. London: HCPC. Available at: www.hcpc-uk.org/globalassets/resources/guidance/guidance-on-conduct-and-ethics-for-students.pdf (accessed November 2022).

Health and Care Professions Council (HCPC) (2017) Standards of education and training. London: HCPC. Available at: www.hcpc-uk.org/globalassets/resources/standards/standards-of-education-and-training.pdf?v=637660865080000000 (accessed November 2022).

Health and Care Professions Council (HCPC) (2018a) Standards of continuing professional development. London: HCPC. Available at: www.hcpc-uk.org/standards/standards-of-continuing-professional-development (accessed November 2022).

Health and Care Professions Council (HCPC) (2018b) Fitness to practise FAQs. London: HCPC. Available at: www.hcpc-uk.org/media-centre/journalist-faqs/fitness-to-practise-faqs (accessed November 2022).

Health and Care Professions Council (HCPC) (2020a) Guidance on the use of social media. London: HCPC. Available at: http://hcpc-uk.org/standards/meeting-our-standards/communication-and-using-social-media/guidance-onuse-of-social-media"hcpc-uk.org/standards/meeting-our-standards/communication-and-using-social-media/guidance-onuse-of-social-media (accessed November 2022).

Health and Care Professions Council (HCPC) (2020b) Our equality, diversity and inclusion strategy 2021–26. London: HCPC. Available at: www.hcpc-uk.org/about-us/equality-diversity-and-inclusion/our-edi-strategy (accessed November 2022).

Health and Care Professions Council (HCPC) (2021a) Consultation on a revised threshold level of qualification for entry to the Register (SET 1) for Operating Department Practitioners (ODPs). London: HCPC. Available at: www.hcpc-uk.org/news-and-events/consultations/2021/consultation-on-a-revised-threshold-level-of-qualification-for-entry-to-the-register-set-1-for-odps (accessed November 2022).

Health and Care Professions Council (HCPC) (2021b) Equality, diversity and inclusion strategy. London: HCPC. Available at: www.hcpc-uk.org/globalassets/meetings-attachments3/council-meeting/2021/23-march-2021/enc-06—equality-diversity-and-inclusion-strategy.pdf (accessed November 2022).

Health and Care Professions Council (HCPC) (2021c) Meeting our standards. London: HCPC. Available at: www.hcpc-uk.org/standards/meeting-our-standards (accessed November 2022).

Health and Care Professions Council (HCPC) (2022) Student hub London: HCPC. Available at: www.hcpc-uk.org/students (accessed November 2022).

Health and Care Professions Council (HCPC) (2023) Standards of proficiency for Operating Department Practitioners. London: HCPC. Available at: https://www.hcpc-uk.org/standards/standards-of-proficiency/operating-department-practitioners/ (accessed November 2022).

Health Education England (HEE) (2017) Multi-professional framework for advanced clinical practice in England. London: HEE. Available at: https://healtheducationengland.sharepoint.com/sites/APWC/Shared%20Documents/   Forms/AllItems.aspx?id=%2Fsites%2FAPWC%2FShared%20Documents%2FHome%2FMulti%2Dprofessional%20framework%20for%20advanced%20clinical%20practice%20in%20England%2Fmulti%2Dprofessionalframeworkforadvancedclinical-practiceinengland%20%281%29%2Epdf&parent=%2Fsites%2FAPWC%2FShared%20Documents%2FHome%2FMulti%2Dprofessional%20framework%20for%20advanced%20clinical%20practice%20in%20England&p=true&ga=1 (accessed July 2023).

Imison, C., Castle-Clark, S. and Watson, R. (2016) Reshaping the workforce to deliver the care patients need: Research report. London: Nuffield Trust.

Macdonald, M.K. (1995) *The Sociology of the Professions*. London: Sage.

McGee, P. (2009) The development of advanced nursing practice in the United Kingdom, in P. McGee (ed.), *Advanced Practice in Nursing and the Allied Health Professions*, 3rd edn. Chichester: Wiley-Blackwell.

National Health Service Executive (NHS Executive) (2000) The employment of Operating Department Practitioners (ODPs): Guidance in the NHS letter dated 20 March 2000. London: NHS Executive.

Nurse Prescribers' Advisory Group (2018) *Nurse Prescribers' Formulary*. London: Pharmaceutical Press.

Saxon, R.L., Gray, M.A. and Oprescu, F.I. (2014) Extended roles for Allied Health Professionals: An updated systematic review of the evidence, *Journal of Multidisciplinary Healthcare*, 7: 479.

Stern, D.T. (ed.) (2006) *Measuring Medical Professionalism*. Oxford: Oxford University Press.

Timmons, S. (2011) Professionalization and its discontents, *Health*, 15(4): 337–52.

Wilkinson, T., Wade, W.B. and Knock, LD. (2009) A blueprint to assess professionalism: Results of a systematic review, *Academic Medicine*, 84: 551–8.

Witz, A. (1992) *Professions and Patriarchy*. Abingdon: Routledge.

Wordsworth, S. (2007) Accountability in peri-operative practice, in B. Smith, P. Rawling, P. Wicker et al. (eds), *Core Topics in Operating Department Practice: Anaesthesia and Critical Care*. Cambridge: Cambridge University Press.

Wordsworth, S. (2014) Professional practice and the Operating Department Practitioner, in H. Abbott and H. Booth (eds), *Foundations for Operating Department Practice: Essential Theory for Practice*. Maidenhead: Open University Press McGraw-Hill Education.

Wordsworth, S. (2015) Student choice in the field of operating department practice, *Journal of Operating Department Practice*, 3(2): 89–95.

Further reading

Legislation

Health Act 1999: www.legislation.gov.uk/ukpga/1999/8/contents (accessed August 2023). (The order was subject to further revocations and amendments in 2003.)

Health and Social Work Order 2001: https://publications.parliament.uk/pa/cm201011/cmbills/132/11132.168-174.html (accessed August 2023).

Health Professions Order 2001: www.legislation.gov.uk/uksi/2002/254/made (accessed August 2023).

Health Professions (Operating Department Practitioners and Miscellaneous Amendments) Order 2004. https://www.legislation.gov.uk/uksi/2004/2033/contents/made (accessed August 2023).

Human Medicines Regulations 2012: https://www.legislation.gov.uk/uksi/2012/1916/contents/made (accessed August 2023).

Human Medicines (Coronavirus and Influenza) (Amendment) Regulations 2020: https://www.legislation.gov.uk/uksi/2020/1125/contents/made (accessed August 2023).

Misuse of Drugs and the Misuse of Drugs (Safe Custody) (Amendment) Regulations 2007: https://www.legislation.gov.uk/uksi/2007/2154/made (accessed August 2023).

4 Operating Department Practitioners (ODPs) working as part of a multidisciplinary team

Hannah Abbott and Helen Booth

Key topics

- How teams and teamworking develop
- The contribution of individual Operating Department Practitioners (ODPs) to their team
- Communication for effective teamworking
- Supervision
- Maintaining your health and well-being

Introduction

The complexity inherent in working in the perioperative environment requires ODPs, who work alongside a wide variety of other professionals, to have highly developed communication and teamworking skills. In addition to these, ODPs need to have a skill set that allows them to manage the range of complex and often stressful situations that present in clinical practice. The aim of this chapter, therefore, is to explore the knowledge and skills that ODPs need to both work in the team and for themselves as individuals in that team, in both perioperative and wider clinical environments.

While communication and teamworking are vast subjects, in this chapter we review some of the key concepts involved and, hopefully, will inspire you to read more about those you find of particular interest. A multidisciplinary team is an organized group of professionals who have developed their knowledge and skills to deliver safe, effective and evidence-based care to their perioperative patients. Therefore, many of the concepts explored in this chapter relate to discussions in other chapters in this book. Any repetition is an indication of how important these topics are to many different aspects of operating department practice and how the fundamental knowledge explored in this text is integral to the care delivered by the perioperative team.

Why is this relevant?

The perioperative environment is a challenging and potentially high-risk one where different healthcare practitioners work together to deliver high-quality care to their patients. To deliver this care, it is essential that ODPs are 'able to work appropriately with others' (Health and Care Professions Council (HCPC) 2023: Standard 8) and must understand the importance of building and sustaining professional relationships as both individual practitioners and collaboratively as members of a team (HCPC 2023). This ability to work effectively in a team has been shown to be essential for patient safety, as poor teamworking behaviours contribute to adverse intraoperative events (Siu et al. 2014) and have been linked to an increased risk of complications or mortality (Mazzocco et al. 2009). Thus, teamworking is included in both the threshold standards for all ODPs and the professional body the College of Operating Department Practitioners' (CODP) pre-registration curriculum, which makes explicit the fundamental need for all ODPs to be able to work effectively in a perioperative team and, hence, in a perioperative environment.

The contributions of individual ODPs to their team

In the perioperative environment, there are various teams:

- the overarching 'perioperative department team';
- teams for specific theatres;
- teams for specific roles, such as the 'anaesthetic team';
- teams for specific shifts, such as the 'late' team.

Many members of staff will belong to more than one team, such as the anaesthetic team and the vascular theatre team, while other teams will be more dynamic – those linked to specific shifts, for example. ODPs also need to be able to work alongside other teams that may come into a theatre and have the ability to work as a new, temporary, team member in other departments, such as when an ODP is required in the emergency department or imaging department.

ODPs, therefore, need to be able to work as individuals in a number of teams and know how to integrate themselves into 'new' teams on a regular basis. To do this effectively, ODPs need to recognize the value of the following two attributes.

Knowledge base and personal experiences

Every team includes several different professionals, each with their own specific knowledge and skills, which is reflected in the roles undertaken by each of them. That there are differentiated but defined roles is another characteristic of a team.

It is crucial, therefore, that ODPs recognize the knowledge that they contribute to the team and how this complements that of their colleagues. It should be remembered that it is not only the knowledge which may vary between professionals but also the underpinning philosophy governing how the knowledge is delivered. For example, there are differences between a traditional 'medical model' of education and a 'nursing model'. The aim of the integration of interprofessional education both pre-and post-registration has been to embed an understanding of other professions so as to improve teamworking and the delivery of care. ODPs should, therefore, seek to maximize these learning opportunities. To work effectively in a team, ODPs need to recognize the value of their own knowledge and be able to assert this confidently while also recognizing the value of others' inputs.

Knowledge, however, is not purely the result of education. Personal experiences result in knowledge, too, and these can have an impact on how practitioners engage with a team regarding a specific case or issue. As we will explore further in the context of evidence-based practice, personal clinical experiences can make a significant contribution to the formation of professional knowledge. Here, however, an important distinction needs to be made between professional experiences, which ODPs can use to inform their practice, and personal experiences, which we have to acknowledge and be able to 'set aside'. That is because personal experiences can have a profound influence on how we perceive a situation and may hamper how a team decision-making process is viewed. ODPs therefore need to be aware of this and able to moderate such influences accordingly. In the same way, an ODP who has had an experience as a patient may feel that their 'service user' view will help the team when delivering care to a patient. However, the ODP would need to consider whether it is professional to share this potentially sensitive information in a team. ODPs must ensure that their interactions in the team, while potentially friendly, must also be professional and sharing information that is personal is both unprofessional and can make other team members very uncomfortable, thus having an adverse impact on the team dynamic.

Confidence and assertiveness

Being confident for ODPs is not only about their knowledge and skill base but also an essential aspect of working in and with teams. Self-confidence is an enabler for ODPs' coping strategies when facing the challenges and problems that arise in operating theatres and related care areas. When confidence requires development, a lack of such coping can reinforce a low level of self-confidence, resulting in a spiraling effect that can have an impact on how the practitioner works in a team. Self-confidence is also important as it enables ODPs to meet the obligation to 'speak up' when poor care is being delivered. This duty was identified as one of the key aspects of NHS England's Patient Safety Strategy (2021).

There is a real need for a supportive environment to be created in a team, as this will contribute to all its members feeling comfortable enough to assert aspects of good practice, concerns and manage any issues effectively. Being able to manage situations well requires assertiveness, which is about being able to express yourself and to speak up not only for your rights but those of patients and others. Being assertive is not about challenging and seeking to dominate or belittle another individual, but is much more about striving to improve, develop and deal with matters effectively as they arise.

It can be difficult to articulate concerns or opinions, but timely communication is paramount in the acute setting of an operating theatre. Not speaking up is to negate ODPs' responsibility to do so and can effectively amount to condoning the observed unacceptable behaviour. Using appropriate skills, ODPs can, for example, handle a situation carefully to ensure that a safety aspect is addressed, behaviour is moderated and others in the team meet and develop compliance with the expected standards.

Multidisciplinary teamworking

There are different definitions of 'team', but they all have some shared characteristics. A team is a group of people who work together or co-ordinate their actions
to achieve a common goal. The perioperative team is known as a 'multidisciplinary' team, which means that it includes individuals with a diverse range of
professional backgrounds. This multidisciplinary nature has been shown to
improve effectiveness and innovation in patient care (Borill et al. 2001). If you
reflect on teams you have been a member of in the past, you will probably think
that this definition would fit most teams. However, it is also important to
think about how teams develop. Many people will have been in teams that they
took an active role in forming, such as when a group of individuals decide to
participate in a team event together. Many people will also have been placed in
an established team – when starting a new job, for example. Effective teams can
be established in both these ways, but it is important for ODPs to understand
more about how teams develop.

Teams in the perioperative environment tend to be dynamic, and shift patterns
dictate that there will be variations in the members of any one team on different
days or for different surgical lists. Consequently, ODPs may be involved in developing teams on a regular basis. Also, teams have to change to accommodate new
members, irrespective of how established those teams are. Hence, there may
often be a period of adjustment for all members when there are such changes to
a team.

Although every team will develop in its own way, an exploration of
teamworking concepts in a number of studies allowed Tuckman (1965) to pro-
pose a model of the usual stages of this process. Tuckman proposed that, initially, the members of a team need to orientate themselves by testing the
boundaries, and this is known as the 'forming' phase. Once a team has formed in
this way, it is inevitable that, as members start to work with one another, there
will be some tensions and conflict. This is known as 'storming', but once these
issues have been resolved, the team will undergo a period of 'norming', during
which they develop their own standards and roles. The final stage in team development is 'performing', which is when the structure supports performance of the
team's role and the members of the team are able to focus their energy on their
task. This model illustrates that all teams have to undergo development and,
hence, ODPs should be prepared for this when working in a new team. It is
important to note that it is not a failing of the team if there are some challenges
as it develops, but it is crucial that these are managed in a professional manner.

Theatre team culture

It is essential that teams recognize the culture they have established and support
new team members as they orientate themselves and settle into the team. In the
same way, new team members need to understand the importance of asking questions when they are unsure, as this will expedite their integration into the team.
As individuals come to know the team and how it works a bit better, they will
become aware of, and embedded in, its unique culture and, while this is generally

welcomed by the individuals, they must be careful that this does not have an adverse impact on their professionalism, such as by them becoming overly familiar in the professional environment.

Irrespective of whether ODPs are established members of a team or new to it, it is important that they recognize how the culture of the team may be perceived by others. If a team has been established for a long time with few changes of staff, its culture may act as a barrier to new team members. This has the potential to pose risks to the patient if the new team member feels that their contributions are unwelcome or they do not feel able to raise a concern. Equally, well-established teams may have developed their own team language, such as calling instruments/ equipment by different names, and this can be confusing for individuals who are new. In such situations, however, individuals must recognize and be prepared to challenge and improve the established culture, to ensure that all staff are valued and supported. It is key to both the staff experience and patient safety that all embrace a culture of improvement and open conversation.

Motivation and shared goals

Having shared goals has been recognized as one of the defining characteristics of teams, the team members then working together to achieve those goals. The aim of achieving the shared goals may therefore be thought of as providing the key motivational driver for the team members to co-ordinate and work effectively to bring them about. This is particularly true of a perioperative team, where the overarching goal is related to the care of the patient, and there is the professional expectation that all team members work towards this. This approach may be in direct contrast to that of some other teams you may have worked in, where there is an element of competition in the team.

Setting goals is also an important part of teamworking, as it is not possible to work together effectively unless all members of the team know what they are working towards. It is often assumed that a perioperative team will have as its shared goals delivering a high standard of care and ensuring that patient safety is optimized. While this will be true for every case, these are fairly generic goals and some cases will benefit from identifying some more specific goals. It is therefore essential that, as part of a team briefing, goals are also identified for individual cases. These goals will be those that are required so as to achieve the overarching goal of safe, high-quality care. For example, in some cases, the priority may be to reduce the overall anaesthetic time. The entire team would need to be aware of this to ensure that any delays on the surgical side are minimized. Alternatively, the goal may be to avoid the need for a blood transfusion, in which case the whole team would need to be aware of the plans made to reduce blood loss.

Attributes that facilitate effective teamworking

Clear, efficient communication is the foundation of playing your part in an effective team and, therefore, a crucial proficiency. Hence, it is Standard 7 in the 'Standards of proficiency: Operating Department Practitioners' (HCPC 2023). It is recognized generally, too, as being paramount to the delivery of effective teamwork. Cited in reports, both in and outside the health service, is the observation that where issues arise at work, they are often down to poor communication, which makes the working environment difficult to manage and means personnel in the team are not working effectively.

As well as communicating effectively, good listening skills are an equally essential part of being an effective team member. It is fundamental that ODPs can follow instructions, co-operate with others and show empathy and understanding to colleagues and those in their care.

Problem-solving skills are valuable in any individual and to a team. This is particularly so in critical situations, when the ability to remain calm and think and act logically to find solutions is a great asset to the team.

The development of critical thinking and collaboration skills through academic activities completed during their studies prepares ODPs for when they need to apply them in a multidisciplinary team. These skills can be used in decision-making, conflict management and giving feedback. Decisions may need to be made at different levels, such as at the individual level or regarding the whole team. At the team level, there are many ways to contribute to making decisions, such as by attending group meetings, talking through matters in a safe environment and being part of a 'for and against' analysis. Critical thinking gives you the ability to look at the facts, evidence and observations and make a judgement informed by evidence.

Conflict management skills and the ability to mediate are invaluable for ensuring the timely resolution of any concerns. Being able to do this is essential in the workplace as, if left unresolved, friction between team members can be disruptive and counterproductive to the delivery of good patient care.

Giving feedback is central to ensuring ongoing improvement and team morale. Consequently, feedback should always be welcome among both team players and superiors. Giving feedback doesn't have to be a negative process, and it is equally important to feed back regarding instances of positive practice too. Constructive criticism can also be an important part of teamwork, however, and it needs to flow in both directions, with all team members being empowered to provide feedback across grades.

Having a positive mindset is an incredibly powerful attribute for teamworking. Positivity is a contagious type of energy – everyone wants to work with colleagues who have such a mindset, as it can inspire people to achieve and result in productive, innovative teams that aspire to excellence in practice. Unfortunately, the opposite is also true. Negativity can adversely affect team morale and culture, and, often, when working with a negative person, you may find that they complain more, won't take responsibility for their own problems and may lack motivation.

Communication for effective practice

In this section, the fundamental theories of communication are not explored, as there are many texts that do this and they are often covered on academic courses. Instead, the focus here is on acknowledging that communication skills are key to ODPs, who also need to understand, develop and reflect on these to see how they can promote better communication throughout their professional life. One thing it is important to realize is that not everyone shares the same preferred communication style. Allen and Brock (2000) cite the Myers–Briggs Type Indicator (MBTI), which is widely used in education and training to understand personality types, and, although each of us is unique, it shows that there are certain behavioural traits that are common to us all and are predictable and consistent.

Communication skills are vital to the role of ODP and, apart from those individuals have naturally, a learned approach should be taken – one that is simple but clear, as it underpins good care. This approach is the foundation of dealing with colleagues, patients and their carers. To communicate effectively, ODPs need to rely on all their skills to not only build trust but also work well with others with the aim of benefiting the patient accessing healthcare. In 2000, Greco et al. identified ten attributes that patients look for in healthcare professionals:

- being greeted warmly;
- being listened to;
- clear explanations;
- reassurance;
- confidence in the ability of the staff;
- able to express their concerns and fears;
- respected;
- given time;
- consideration given to personal circumstances when seeking advice or treatment;
- being treated like a person and not what they clinically present with.

These aspects are still important to patients, as can seen from many reports in which patients have raised concerns.

ODPs play a significant role in managing the messages given to patients and others as part of the perioperative team. In the perioperative environment, there are many factors that affect the flow of information, such as interruptions, team familiarity, unpredictable incidents and changes to schedules. Where errors have occurred, the root cause cited in many cases has been communication failures. To improve communication, briefings and time out have been developed and since become a part of the perioperative preparation routine.

There are three related aspects that affect communication in a team in an operating theatre, which are the:

- nature of the task that needs to be done;
- procedure followed to ensure the task is performed effectively;
- interpersonal relationships between those in the team.

Related to these, there are some unavoidable barriers that affect communication in the perioperative environment. One of these is the wearing of hats and surgical masks, which can create difficulty in hearing the message, distort it or even lead to misinterpretation because, for example, the listener is unable to see the speaker's lips move. Medical and other specialist terminology can also be a barrier. This is frequently used by those who work in perioperative teams for various types of swabs, for example, plus abbreviations and acronyms, that are like some kind of code, which alienate those who are not familiar with them. Cultural variations in language can also contribute to forming a barrier to a message being received and transmitted correctly, so ODPs need to be aware of the impact of cultural considerations on communication. ODPs will also recognize how team dynamics play an important role in setting the scene for the surgical procedure and the care to be delivered. The theatre environment is generally quiet but there are sources of noise that can interfere with how a message is transmitted and received. For example, some surgeons or patients who are awake may wish to have music playing and there are noises that come from the technology and equipment used, such as ventilators, monitors, suction, and surgical equipment, such as power tools, and these can all distort or interfere with communication.

It is equally important to communicate messages effectively when providing written records of care for patients, when receiving them and when transferring their care to others in the perioperative environment. All records should be clear and legible, using no jargon and ensuring that those who will receive the information will understand it correctly. Abbreviations are to be avoided unless they are recognized terminology used by all. This is crucial, particularly when a patient is being moved from one care setting to another. The quality and continuity of care provided by the many teams the patient will come into contact with relies heavily on the interpersonal skills and the effective sharing of appropriate information, both verbally and through the written records of care.

Patients' views of their care will be affected by the interpersonal skills of the ODPs looking after them and the interactions they have with them. Non-verbal communication is just as important as the words spoken, sometimes more so. Gestures used can be discouraging for patients, especially when, for example, they are greeted by someone who, during the anaesthetic phase, leans against the workstation with folded arms, thus giving the message of not being bothered about them. Likewise, members of the team dashing about can relay the message to patients that they are very busy, maybe too busy to speak to them, and so patients may neglect to ask questions or share important information, feeling that they do not want to 'be a burden' or 'bother' an already busy team. Teams need to recognize these kinds of issues and raise them in the appropriate forum so that they can put in place more patient-sensitive modes of behaviour in the perioperative environment.

Teams need to look at their approaches to all these and other areas of communication and consider the potential impacts these can have on not only patients but also members of staff, in whatever capacity they are working, who can be equally affected.

Active listening

The term 'active listening' is often used by healthcare professionals to stress the importance of the need to listen, and not merely to the words being spoken but also to the many complex layers of meaning that the person speaking is relaying to you.

The nature of the skill of listening will vary depending on the context and the matter in hand. In an operating theatre, for example, an ODP may need to elicit important information that is crucial to the task in hand, whether this is taking down vital signs to be reported to another or gathering patient-specific information to be used in their care. A good questioning technique can be supportive of active listening, such as using open or closed questions, which will encourage a certain response depending on the information needed. Using this can support other tools in achieving effective communication.

Stop and think

Have you noticed how communication has changed since it has become common-place to have online video calls via Teams or Zoom? As some patient interactions, such as a pre-assessment, are delivered online, how can you ensure that you communicate effectively via an online conversation?

You might want to consider how you can convey that you are listening to the patient, how your body language comes across online and how you can avoid distraction.

Using the SBAR tool to aid communication in the perioperative team

The dynamic nature of the clinical environment and interventions means that information must be communicated effectively. For example, when ODPs are caring for patients, they may exhibit a rapid change in their physiological state, both during and after surgery. Consequently, ODPs need to be able to identify that there is cause for concern and raise this effectively and in a timely manner. It is therefore essential that all relevant information is handed over to other practitioners in the team, especially if there are any concerns, and these are communicated effectively.

To support ODPs as they do this, the National Health Service (NHS) Institute for Innovation and Improvement (2010) advocates the use of the SBAR tool, which stands for situation, background, assessment and recommendation. It provides a structure to ensure that the essential information is shared in a clear and concise way. It can be used to inform verbal or written communications at any point in the patient journey. The steps taken when using SBAR for communications are as follows and an example of an ODP raising a concern with a medic regarding a patient in the post-anaesthetic care unit (PACU) is shown in Table 4.1.

- **Situation:** The ODP should initially describe the situation. This includes identifying yourself, which is particularly important in the perioperative environment when all staff wear the same medical scrubs and even though you may 'know' another colleague on a conversational basis, they may not be aware of your professional background. The situation also needs to include an explanation of who the patient is and the cause for concern.
- **Background:** This will help the reader or listener to gain a full picture of the patient, especially as you may be talking to a member of the on-call surgical team rather than someone from the team that operated on the patient. When explaining the patient's background, include why the patient was admitted and relevant medical history. This is important so that the recipient can start to consider the situation and so allows conversation about the patient to be more effective. If in person, in an environment where there are time pressures, all

practitioners should aim to make each conversation effective. For example, there would be no value in describing a case and a medic issuing a verbal prescription to then be told that the patient is allergic to that drug, so including all such information at this stage allows the recipient to start to build a complete picture from the salient information about the patient.

- **Assessment:** In this stage, the ODP reports their assessment of the case, including vital signs and a clinical assessment. The ODP should have come to this assessment as a result of considering other objective measures and the potential cause for concern. This demonstrates the need for ODPs to have good skills for assessing patients and a comprehensive understanding of anatomy and physiology.
- **Recommendation:** The final stage requires the ODP to make a recommendation. This is not specifically for clinical care but, rather, it is what you need to achieve by the end of the conversation. This may be instructions for what actions the ODP needs to take, which may be to prepare equipment or receive a verbal prescription. To make this recommendation, the ODP needs to be clear about what they require from the other person and should end the conversation or notes with clearly agreed actions.

The SBAR tool is a structured way to share necessary information effectively with other team members, the four stages including all that it is important to know for any handover. The example given in Table 4.1 is of SBAR being used in a telephone conversation to raise a concern about a deteriorating patient and it shows how the key information can be communicated succinctly to brief another professional on the patient's clinical condition. The four stages of the SBAR can be applied equally effectively to other situations and modes of communication, however, as it always ensures that the salient information is included. ODPs should therefore ensure that they are familiar with this tool.

Stop and think

Could you use this SBAR to ensure you communicate all relevant information in other handovers? For example at shift change – you may want to think about using the recommendations to explain what is still needed. Try to write an SBAR in the anaesthetic role when handing over a patient undergoing a complex procedure to the next shift.

Supervision

The fundamental desire of any ODP is to ensure that they improve and develop their practice through research, reflection and active participation in their learning. In March 2020 the HCPC developed resources that broaden the term 'supervision' in relation to such development, covering a wider range of what this may be. It now covers practice/clinical supervision, professional supervision and operational/line management supervision. Essentially, therefore, it is there to

Table 4.1 Example of the SBAR tool in practice

	Example of SBAR in use	*Context*
Situation	'This is ODP Alexa Berry from the post-anaesthetic care unit in main theatres. I am calling about Mrs Kelly from the gynaecology list this afternoon. She has been in PACU for 1 hour and has become increasingly tachycardic, she is also tachypneic and hypotensive.'	This concise summary immediately informs the other person who they are speaking to and the reason for the call and has therefore 'set the scene' for the conversation that follows.
Background	'Mrs Kelly is a 45-year-old woman who was admitted this morning for an elective vaginal hysterectomy. She had a spinal anaesthetic and it is noted that she was a potentially difficult intubation. All her pre-operative investigations were normal and she has no allergies. She was on hormone replacement therapy that she stopped 4 weeks before surgery.'	The ODP has provided a summary of all the relevant medical history. The medic now knows that Mrs Kelly was otherwise fit and well and, should she need to return to theatre, there is the potential that she will be difficult to intubate.
Assessment	'Mrs Kelly is tachycardic with a weak, thready pulse of 110 beats per minute, her blood pressure is 75/50 mmHG, her respiration rate is 28, she has not produced any urine in the last hour and she is cool and clammy to the touch. She is exhibiting signs of hypovolaemic shock and I think she might be bleeding internally.'	This assessment has clearly indicated the severity of Mrs Kelly's condition and the ODP has offered a suggestion as to what she believes the cause may be, based on her clinical assessment.
Recommendation	'I think you need to come and see Mrs Kelly. How soon can you get here? Would you like me to order blood products/ arrange for the emergency theatre to be on standby?'	The ODP has said what she requires (the medic to review Mrs Kelly) and has asked for an indication of when the medic will be arriving and what can be done in the interim to prepare for the subsequent care of the patient, based on the presentation and initial assessment.

support all aspects of professional development. ODPs who embrace supervision of their practice will see it as another tool of lifelong learning and an invaluable way to demonstrate their professional responsibility and accountability.

The resources dovetail with the 'Standards of proficiency' (HCPC 2023: 4.8) and 'Standards of conduct, performance and ethics' (HCPC 2016: 2.5), and the HCPC (2021) states that, 'while there is no single or agreed definition of supervision, at its core, supervision is a process of professional learning and development that enables individuals to reflect on and develop their knowledge, skills, and competence, through agreed and regular support with another professional'. Though it may take a variety of forms – managerial, clinical or professional, for example – the essence of the concept is to review performance, discuss cases or objectives or look at development. Supervision also sets out training needs, any modification of practice or levels of compliance with professional conduct and codes.

The focus for the majority of ODPs will be on clinical supervision, as this addresses both the professional and personal aspects for those working in the perioperative environment, although the other forms of supervision may have an impact on the overall outcome. As a profession, ODPs have not yet formalized their approach towards clinical supervision, but it has advantages for registered professionals, who need to meet set standards, such as the regulatory standards.

ODPs who are in advanced roles working in places other than theatres and with wider multidisciplinary teams may already be familiar with supervision. However, at the time of writing, it is still in the early stages of development for those working in theatres. To ensure that the supervision is effective, therefore, it is important that a safe and confidential process is developed in the perioperative environment to support and develop ODPs and their colleagues to discuss and express opinions on aspects of their work and how they can improve or develop these further. The benefits of developing the process of supervision in the perioperative environment are threefold.

- The individual ODP can benefit as it will enable them to reflect on, discuss and develop, as well as challenge their own practice, gain feedback from peers and contribute to their professional development. It complements the continuing professional development requirements of the regulator and provides ODPs with new avenues for developing that can be achieved by working with others.
- The whole team benefits by gaining a sense of value and the chance to develop a shared culture in which to work. This works best if there is an established benchmark of behaviours and openness to identify skill deficits in a team and how a greater understanding of one another's roles and responsibilities can improve the working practices of all. It also enables those who feel that they need or want more support to express this and discuss how this can be achieved and shared in the team in a non-judgemental, safe environment.
- Ultimately, the patients who come to an operating theatre benefit the most from supervision as they will receive high-quality care, as the ultimate aim of clinical supervision is the improvement of practice. The patient will also be cared for by staff who are supportive of one another and are able to manage the emotional, personal and professional aspects of their practice and thus are a more effective team.

The most effective approaches or models for supervision are when it takes place either one to one or in a group. The one-to-one methods, as mentioned, will be more familiar to those working in operating theatres, particularly newly qualified practitioners. The successful supervision of newly qualified practitioners will lead to an increase in confidence in their ability to understand and learn the responsibilities of their role, help with the challenges at this stage in their professional development and assure them that there is a robust support structure. To ensure that the process is effective, however, it is advised not to use one method only without exploring the others.

When the supervision begins, it should be made clear that it is all about support and development; it is not a covert way to manage someone's performance. There are other tools available for doing that. Supervision is about using the right approach to manage each situation. It is also important to set expectations and establish ground rules, the most important of these relating to honesty and trust, which must be maintained at all times. The focus needs to be on creating a safe environment that allows ODPs to reflect on and develop their practice without feeling that it is always subject to scrutiny. The supervision process relies on establishing good relationships between the supervisor and those they are supervising.

The supervisor should have appropriate qualifications, knowledge and skills in the area of practice that they will be supervising. In addition, they need to have the essential non-technical skills, such as good interpersonal and problem-solving skills, and be able to give effective and timely feedback. The supervisor should also be a role model, maintaining their own professional development and seeking supervision of their practice and the roles that they are undertaking.

The supervisor needs to be clear about the type or model of supervision that they will be embarking on with the individual or group. It is important that they are supportive and approachable, aware of the individuals' or group's experience and skills, identify their personal and professional development needs, keep records of the sessions and review any plans made, ensuring that they are actioned in the specified time. Both the supervisor and supervised need to understand that any issues arising regarding concerns about conduct, competence and health of an ODP will need to be shared and managed appropriately, which may be outside the supervision process.

ODPs undertaking supervision should be active rather than passive and, hence, should prepare for the sessions by identifying areas of their practice that they wish to discuss. They should keep records of their sessions and take responsibility for completing the agreed actions, which could form part of what needs to be discussed further at development reviews or appraisals.

Stop and think

What areas of your practice would you like to discuss openly on a one-to-one basis or in a group that would benefit your personal and professional development and the care you provide to patients?

Supporting health and well-being in operating department practice

The NHS's People Promise is a key component of the NHS England's 'We are the NHS: People Plan 2020/21' (2020), which recognizes the diversity of the NHS workforce and the importance of the 1.3 million people who make up the organization. The COVID-19 pandemic raised awareness of the importance of and need for ODPs to take care of themselves so that they can deliver the best care and, hence, the aim of the People Promise is to build on the learning from the pandemic. There was significant work completed during it, to offer additional support services to all healthcare staff, including dedicated confidential support, access to mental health and well-being resources and additional support for line managers. The intention is that the NHS will continue to develop and build on the practical and emotional support offered and, as a result, the employers' offer should include (NHS England 2020):

- a well-being guardian in the organization;
- safe spaces where staff can rest and recuperate;
- psychological support and treatment;
- physically heathy work environments;
- support to 'switch off' from work, to decrease the risk of work-related stress.

It is important that ODPs embrace the ethos of the People Promise, both for their own well-being and that of their colleagues. This is reflected in the updated Standards of proficiency, which require registrants to 'look after their health and wellbeing, seeking appropriate support where necessary' (HCPC 2023: Standard 8), which includes both physical and mental health in addition to recognizing stress and anxiety in themselves. As part of collegiate teams in the perioperative environment, ODPs have the opportunity to support their colleagues' well-being and initiate a conversation when they suspect someone is struggling. While these are potentially difficult to initiate, they can have a significant impact and sometimes simply taking the time to ask if someone is okay (and really listening to the answer) is the first step to accessing support.

There are health and well-being resources available and some key documents can be found online, such as:

- NHS England – has pages supporting staff health and well-being;
- Association of Anaesthetists – its well-being and support pages have a wealth of resources, including ones related to fatigue after working night shifts.

Recognizing and managing stress in practice

ODPs encounter stressful situations in their work and so need to develop effective mechanisms to identify and manage their stress. Stressful situations may manifest from a number of triggers in a team. For example, they could relate to technical equipment, personal or patient-related problems, teamwork issues, distractions and difficulty with time management. Stress may also arise from other factors such as a death in the perioperative environment or the highly emotional aspect of caring for terminally ill children who come in to the operating theatre. A lot of these situations are not under the control of ODPs and can have a significant impact on the performance of the individual and the team. While patient safety is paramount and technical skills are developed to a high level, these are not the only factors that ODPs should consider as part of their role.

It is worth noting at this point that it is often the non-technical skills of communication, awareness of the situation, leadership and poor decision-making skills that can lead to poor outcomes for patients. Thus, ODPs must be able to identify their own stress and its potential impact on their practice (HCPC 2023: Standard 3.1). This is an important part of being a professional as the more stressed an individual becomes, the greater is the risk that they will make a mistake. It can be hard for ODPs to recognize stress in themselves, as it can manifest in a variety of ways. However, if it continues for a long period, it can cause psychological, mental and physical symptoms. The causes of stress can be related to the demand of the workload and lack of control in expressing this. It could be a lack of support or changes to your role or the environment and those you work with. Equally, stress can come from personal problems, finances, bereavement, divorce, childcare difficulties, moving house and a wide variety of health issues, either personally or related to a relationship.

Stressful situations in the operating theatre should not always be viewed as negative as ODPs may find that an individual acutely stressful situation, such as an emergency case, enables them to work particularly effectively. However, debriefing from these stressful cases is important, both as a valuable learning event and as an opportunity to help both the team and individual manage these stressful times better in the future. The impact of day-to-day-stress, such as workload, needs to be managed by ODPs to ensure that it does not adversely affect their well-being.

ODPs, therefore, need to be aware of the signs of stress and know what actions to take, especially if their stress is exacerbated by their work. In addition to the NHS resources previously discussed, ODPs may also seek support via their line manager or general practitioner. For student ODPs, there are support services available via their university and their personal tutor or link tutor is a good starting point for signposting them to the available services.

Recognizing the early signs of stress is important, as being able to do this will help to prevent it getting worse and leading to further health problems. ODPs' health is paramount when dealing with patients and so being able to manage their stress is a crucial aspect of fulfilling their professional responsibility. It is ODPs' responsibility to ensure that they discuss such matters at an early stage with their line manager or personal tutor.

Stop and think

Think about an occasion when you experienced a period of tension or stress. This may have been when you had a number of deadlines to meet, a number of personal issues in addition to your work or maybe a very high-pressure event.

Think about how you knew you were stressed. How did those signs of stress manifest? What could have been the potential impact on your practice of this stress?

Now think about what you did or could have done to rectify this.

Do you know where to find support services? If not, take some time to explore what is available to you and your colleagues.

Conclusion

This chapter has explored the many facets of working in a multidisciplinary team and the complexity of teams that are dynamic and, hence, constantly evolving and developing. This constant development process requires ODPs to be adaptive members of their team, able to modify their behaviour to integrate themselves into it, while retaining their professional identify and asserting their professional knowledge. To achieve this effectively, ODPs need a good level of self-awareness, so they can recognize both their input to the team and those of others. The focus of the perioperative team will always be on the delivery of high-quality care to patients and, therefore, the team needs to ensure that the specific goals to achieve this are articulated and agreed. It is essential to do this to enable the team as a whole, and hence ODPs, to work effectively towards its shared goal.

Key points

- To work effectively, teams must have a clear goal that has been agreed by the team.
- Effective communication is a vital component of professional responsibility and ODPs need to be able to recognize the barriers to this and address them appropriately.
- Professional well-being is paramount to being an effective practitioner, caring for those in their care.
- Supervision can provide support to and develop ODPs as part of their ongoing professional development.

References and further reading

Allen, J. and Brock, S.A. (2000) *Healthcare Communication Using Personality Type*. Abingdon: Routledge.

Borill, C.S., Carletta, J., Carter, A.J., et al. (2001) The effectiveness of health care teams in the National Health Service: Report. Birmingham: University of Aston. Available at: www.researchgate.net/publication/238686262_The_Effectiveness_of_Health_Care_Teams_in_the_National_Health_Service_Report (accessed November 2022).

Greco, M., Brownlea, A., McGovern, J., et al. (2000) Consumers as educators: Implementation of patient feedback in general practice training, *Health Communications*, 12(1): 73–93.

Health and Care Professions Council (HCPC) (2016) Standards of conduct, performance and ethics. London: HCPC. Available at: www.hcpc-uk.org/standards/standards-of-conduct-performance-and-ethics (accessed November 2022).

Health and Care Professions Council (HCPC) (2021) Supervision: Reflect, discuss, develop: The benefits of supervision. London: HCPC. Available at: www.hcpc-uk.org/standards/meeting-our-standards/supervision-leadership-and-culture/supervision (accessed November 2022).

Health and Care Professions Council (HCPC) (2023) Standards of proficiency: Operating Department Practitioners. London: HCPC. Available at: https://www.hcpc-uk.org/globalassets/resources/standards/standards-of-proficiency---odp.pdf?v=637106257360000000 (accessed November 2022).

Mazzocco K., Petitti D.B., Fong K.T., et al. (2009) Surgical team behaviours and patient outcomes, *American Journal of Surgery*, 197: 678–85.

National Health Service (NHS) Institute for Innovation and Improvement (2010) Safer care: SBAR: Situation Background Assessment Recommendation: Implementation and training guide. London: NHS Institute for Innovation and Improvement. Available at: www.england. nhs.uk/improvement-hub/wp-content/uploads/sites/44/2017/11/SBAR-Implementation-and-Training-Guide.pdf (accessed November 2022).

NHS England (2020) We are the NHS: People Plan 2020/21: Action for us all. London: NHS England. Available at: www.england.nhs.uk/wp-content/uploads/2020/07/We-Are-The-NHS-Action-For-All-Of-Us-FINAL-March-21.pdf (accessed November 2022).

NHS England (2021) The NHS Patient Safety Strategy. London: NHS England. Available at: www. england.nhs.uk/patient-safety/the-nhs-patient-safety-strategy (accessed July 2023).

Siu, J., Maran, N. and Paterson-Brown, S. (2014) Observation of behavioural markers of non-technical skills in the operating room and their relationship to intra-operative incidents, *Surgeon*, 14(3): 119–28.

Tuckman, B. (1965) Developmental sequence in small groups, *Psychological Bulletin*, 63(6): 3.

5 | Reflection for Operating Department Practitioners

Penny Joyce

Key topics

- Reflection in operating department practice
- Reflective practice as an everyday occurrence
- Reflective professional practice
- Types of reflection – reflection on and in action
- Ways to reflect
- The consequences of reflection
- Toolkit for reflection

Introduction

Reflection is an important human activity in which people recapture an experience, think about it, mull ideas over and evaluate it. It is this working with an experience that is important in learning (Boud et al. 1985: 43).

Reflection is an integral part of our lives, as a student Operating Department Practitioner (ODP), an experienced practitioner or simply as part of everyday activities. It is more than a buzzword – it presents an opportunity to draw your thoughts together, gives focus and demonstrates learning. Frequently used in education with a structured approach, it allows students to move from a simple descriptive framework to more complex processes that allow deeper, more critical thinking. When used more informally, it is part of everyday activities, human development and interactions.

In this chapter, the relevance of reflection to learners is explored. This includes pre-registration students but also acknowledges that at any stage in our career we are all learners to some degree, so must consider the opportunities and tools for learning through reflection, reflective writing, professional development and the more analytical and critical aspects of reflection. References will be made to the literature as it includes seminal texts that still underpin much of the evidence base that is relevant today.

Without doubt, reflection is seen as an essential component in improving professional practice for health professionals. Schön (1983) is a name synonymous with reflection in healthcare, but he was not the first to provide evidence for its benefits. In fact, Schön did not write about healthcare professionals in particular but he, along with Boud et al. (1985) and Dewey (1933), has been among the most influential in developing the use of reflection in healthcare education, particularly in nursing (Jasper 2003). Schön remains at the core of contemporary thinking in relation to professionals' application of reflective action and thinking. The significance of his work still influences many training and education programmes, with the philosophy of theory and practice being tightly integrated as a core component.

Dewey (1933) defined 'reflection' as an active, persistent and careful consideration of any belief or supposed form of knowledge in the light of the grounds that support it and the further conclusion it reaches. Boud et al. (1985) have a different perspective, defining it as more of a generic term for those intellectual and effective activities individuals engage in to explore their experiences to lead to new understandings and appreciation of them. They view reflection from the learner's point of view, discussing the relationship of the reflective process and the learning experience to what the learner can do.

Why is this relevant?

The Health and Care Professions Council (HCPC 2023), through the 'Standards of proficiency for Operating Department Practitioners', and the College of Operating Department Practitioners (CODP), which clearly articulates the use of reflection in the professional curriculum, both promote the need for reflection and the ability to reflect as key outcomes for ODPs (CODP 2018: 15, 21, 23) as a means for developing and promoting safe and effective patient care. The recommendations from the report 'Gross negligence manslaughter in healthcare' (Williams 2018) included raising the profile and value of reflection, which are vital to both learning and improving patient care. In a small-scale ODP cohort study, it was shown that student learning is reliant on an experiential approach (in this case it was simulation) and reflection is a vehicle for effecting cognitive change (Joyce 2011).

ODPs need to develop strong interpersonal skills to facilitate patient care in the operating theatre environment. This, together with self-awareness and the ability to directly influence or change practice to ensure positive outcomes in all aspects of perioperative care, are key skills. Reflective practice facilitates the development of these key skills by encouraging ODPs to understand the events or experiences that happen and, of them, through analysis, come to a deeper understanding or clarity about them, which can be used to inform future and evolving practice.

> Reflection is the thought process where individuals consider their experiences to gain insights about their whole practice. Reflection supports individuals to continually improve the way they work or the quality of care they give to people. It is a familiar, continuous and routine part of the work of health and care professionals.

This quote, from a statement by all nine of the healthcare regulators, including the HCPC, supporting healthcare practitioners becoming reflective practitioners (HCPC 2019: 1), further reinforces the relevance of reflection to ODPs. The statement clearly sets out the commitment of all the regulators to reflection and recognizes the role it plays in teams for developing ideas and improving practice. Following the Williams report (2018), each of the regulators set out its requirements for registrants and, for ODPs, this relates to standards for continuing professional development (CPD; HCPC 2017). The HCPC (2017: 4) notes, 'developing evidence suggests that the most effective learning activities are often those that are interactive and which encourage self-reflection'. In addition, the 'Standards of proficiency: Operating Department Practitioners' (HCPC 2023) require registrants to engage in and understand the value of reflection and record their reflections.

Stop and think

Think about some of the everyday experiences you have had in the past few weeks, such as washing your laundry, shopping, socializing, reading, driving, eating and going to work or where you are a student. Now ask yourself the questions in the bulleted list in the section under the heading 'Reflective practice as an everyday occurrence'. Have you considered these questions, which you may ask yourself during everyday activities, as a process of reflective learning?

Reflective practice as an everyday occurrence

The professional and regulatory position is clear: this topic is relevant to ODPs, as both learners and practitioners, and reflection is simply embedded in everyday life. 'Experiences' happen all the time, consciously and subconsciously. We think about what happened and 'relive' an experience, even if we do this later or do not take it any further than it being simply a descriptive process. However, we rarely take the time to analyse the routine and everyday experiences we have and ask ourselves questions about them.

- What have I just done or experienced?
- Why did I do it that way?
- Have I done it before – did the last time influence me this time?
- Could I have done it any differently?
- How will I do it next time?

Take the example of 'washing your laundry' in the case of a student who is currently living away from home at university. This is their first experience of selecting products such as washing powder, liquid or fabric softener. When reflecting on the brand of washing powder they chose, they said that they picked the same brand that they had seen being used at home, which was considered 'very good'. Their choice, therefore, was influenced by a previous experience. The student could have bought any brand, maybe gone for the cheapest, biggest pack or best value for money. These are all aspects that may influence the student in the future.

This experience could apply to many everyday aspects of life – the bread we buy, the beer we drink or the drive to work – but we do not have the time to sit back and reflect in a structured way on every routine experience we have. Jasper (1999) explains this process as having three components that make up the cycle of experience, reflection and action, and presents a very simple framework for reflection that suggests we learn from thinking about things that have happened to us. This applies equally to both everyday life and developing our professional practice.

The process of managing 'routine' experiences makes us effective and time efficient in our daily activities, but as we gain experience and watch others, by observing things done differently, we will begin to change the ways we do things. Even if, after experimenting by trying these, we revert to the way we have always done them, that decision will be based on reflective thinking and reflective practice, albeit from a passive stance.

Learners demonstrate learning through reflection, and it is a tool they are introduced to early in their education. Johns (1995) notes that reflection enables practitioners to assess, understand and learn through their experiences. The development of professional expertise is more than a collection of knowledge and skills; it is the integration of knowledge and skills appropriate to each unique situation that is faced (Eraut 1994). It is a personal process that usually results in some change in their perspective on a situation or creates new learning.

The connection between reflection and learning has been developed by a number of educational theorists, but one who is key and the most well-known is Kolb (1984). His work on the experiential learning cycle (see Figure 5.1) has been the foundation of many other models for reflective practice. Kolb's theory directs us to recall and observe an experience we want to learn from, reflect on that experience and, in so doing, describe the experience. Once described, you can then try to make sense of it (analyse) – what happened, why it happened – and, perhaps explore other theories relating to the experience (read around the subject, look at the evidence base, for example) and work out your own theories or ideas about it. This process will allow you to gain a greater understanding and, as Kolb proposes, help you to frame some future action – that action being the result of learning.

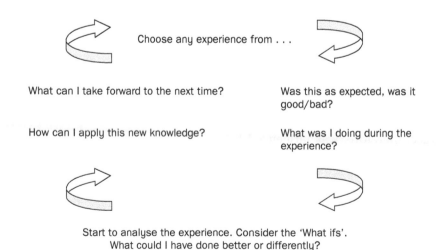

Figure 5.1 Learning from experiences

Source: Adapted from Kolb (1984)

Kolb (1984) proposes four phases of experiential learning, which are essentially reflective:

1 the experience;
2 reflection on what has happened – 'Was it a good, poor or mediocre performance?', 'What did I learn from the experience – I know what I am doing or need to learn more?';
3 'abstract conceptualization', which is when the student will attempt to understand why they went wrong or did well or could have improved and start to consider, 'Next time, I'll . . .';
4 application of the knowledge or skills learnt from the experience.

Of course, this is a cyclical process, so it never really comes to an end – it simply continues to evolve as the lifelong learner does, with each new experience, knowledge and theory increasing their learning as they go through each revolution of the cycle. Therefore, reflection is associated with a deep approach to learning that allows for new information to be integrated with existing knowledge and skills.

Sandars (2009: 693) identified that reflection was often not integrated into the curriculum, seen as a 'bolt on extra'. In such a situation, both tutors and students are in danger of seeing it as being disconnected from the learning process on their courses, which can result in poor engagement and (this is considered in relation to a consequence of reflection later in this chapter).

For professional practice, this cycle of learning is essential to developing our role as ODPs – the learning from our experiences is constantly being fed back into our practice and building our knowledge and experience every time. This learning process, therefore, is not just looking back but is a spiral of learning that moves into the future, as experience develops, facilitating planning for further development and new experiences.

Stop and think

Think back to an event, good or bad.

Why this event? Why is it significant to you?

Has it made an impact on any further similar experiences or will it factor in any future events?

Reflective professional practice

Reflection places value on an experience and offers the opportunity to show where learning and changes have taken place. This will encourage you to pose and answer key questions about your future experiences, such as, 'Why did it happen, when did it happen and how did it happen?'. Doing so gives you an opportunity to place your experiences in the context of your professional practice and to record the learning that comes out of such experiences, whether you are a student or qualified ODP, and at any stage in the development of your career. An important aspect of becoming or being a practitioner is developing the ability to reflect on everyday experiences in a meaningful way and in a variety of settings. You might choose to reflect to:

- consider practices as part of your continuing professional development;
- learn from specific incidents;
- share good practice;
- develop new ideas;
- identify personal learning needs;
- learn a new task, skill or technique;
- explore personal feelings;
- make sense of an incident or experience;
- demonstrate an ability to others;
- problem-solve;
- support decision-making;
- debrief yourself and others;
- anticipate (by reflecting before taking action).

These are just some areas that can benefit from reflection – this list is not exhaustive – but clearly reflective practice provides a key framework for practitioners and aspiring practitioners to learn from their experiences. In the perioperative environment, the last use of reflection listed – to anticipate – is a key skill. For example, when assisting with a potentially difficult airway, an ODP may reflect on similar previous experiences to inform their actions.

The notion of 'experience' is worth considering here. There is often a tendency to consider an experience 'critical' in terms of its complexity, urgency or consequence, but any life event, however routine and simple, can contribute to development. This can be the case whether the outcomes of such events have been positive, negative or completely neutral. It may also be so whether it was a series of events or an accumulation of experience over time. So 'experience' should be thought of in its broadest sense – it could well be a one-off event, a process over time, skills or knowledge. The trigger for reflection can be an experience that:

- have gone really well;
- went badly wrong;
- you did not understand;
- you feel really good about;
- made you feel uncomfortable or sad or angry;
- you received feedback on regarding your role in it or your performance;
- you want to share with others.

It can be seen from this that reflective practice carries multiple meanings, both in terms of why you reflect and what you reflect on. The reasons for the choices made will always be individual and, as a learner or practitioner, the more formal and structured approaches are usually determined by explicit criteria in the curriculum being followed. Smyth (1992: 285) suggests that 'reflection can mean all things to all people . . . it is used as a kind of umbrella or canopy term to signify something is good or desirable'.

There is a danger for learners and practitioners that reflection can become a ritual, sometimes artificial in the desire to ensure that professional and regulatory bodies' criteria to be a 'reflective practitioner' are met. Practices such as a checklist for reflection on practice placements, for example, can be mechanistic and lead learners and practitioners to be unaware of the consequences of reflection at times.

The consequences of reflection

As we have seen, reflective practice is widely acknowledged to be an essential foundation for professional development and a tool for lifelong learning. Done well, it is a valuable tool to explore, transform and progress practice, but it also raises some consequences, which need to be considered whether you are a registered ODP, a student or delivering ODP education.

Teaching reflective practice raises two main concerns: first, the extent to which students are ready, in terms of their development, to reflect appropriately; and, second, mandatory reflective practice, by virtue of a pre-registration curriculum, for example. A readiness to reflect can be problematic as learners, by their nature, are novices in their chosen professional field, so movement from the descriptive stage to the action (learning) stage needs to be carefully nurtured. Often, learners are not aware of the issues that need to be considered at the evaluation stage. If they are presented only with a checklist on which to reflect their learning from practice experience, what will happen is that it will become process-driven and they will not develop the skills to consider what, why and how to reflect on any given experience. Finlay (2008: 16) suggests the following four guiding principles for educators:

- present reflective practice with care;
- provide adequate support, time, resources, opportunities and methods for reflection;
- develop (learners') skills of critical analysis;
- take proper account of the context for reflection.

The mandatory requirement that reflection be included in an ODP pre-registration programme has the potential to make the process very false. It has been found that learners from other professions where the assessment of reflection is significant adopt an approach to perform it in a certain way simply to achieve a pass (Hargreaves 2004). Hobbs (2007: 413) makes a more radical suggestion, that 'reflection and assessment are incompatible'. However, even with academically driven activities, such as 'having to do reflection', it is still widely acknowledged as being valuable for deepening understanding.

Professional and ethical consequences are other aspects to be considered. Some of the ethical issues relate to confidentiality, informed consent, professional relationships, disclosure, misconduct, status of the records (if reflections are written or recorded) and the emotional impact.

As important as learning about the ways in which to reflect and models for reflection, therefore, is to share the wider context of the possible risks and ensure that students are fully aware of the potential for conflicts of interest. Reflection can have a profound emotional effect on the reflector, so it is essential to be aware that this carries a risk of causing harm.

However, it is also the case that an essential component of emotional well-being is understanding your thoughts and feelings, and self-reflection is a positive way to manage this. Healthcare is an ever-changing, stressful and dynamic environment and ODPs may well find themselves working outside their level of expertise, so they need to ensure that, when necessary, they refer the situation to an appropriate practitioner or expert (HCPC 2023). Resilience is not about being self-sufficient; it can be a very resilient act to seek help when you need it.

Stop and think

Think of an event or issue that concerned you.

What were your feelings?

Did you or could you have asked for help?

Analyse all negative thoughts or feelings – are they valid?

Types of reflection – reflection on and in action

Schön (1983), who remains one of the most influential writers on this topic, describes reflection in two main ways: as reflection *on* action and reflection *in* action. Reflection *on* action is looking back after the event, while reflection *in* action is happening during the event. In professional practice, examples of reflecting on practice are thinking about an experience after it happened, judging how successful it was, what you could do better and so on. Fitzgerald (1994: 67) defines this as 'the retrospective contemplation of practice undertaken in order to uncover the knowledge used in practical situations, by analysing and interpreting the information recalled'.

This is the most common type of reflection student ODPs engage in as part of their studies and knowledge development, and for those new to reflection, this is also usually the starting point.

Reflection *in* action allows an ODP to redesign what they are doing while they are doing it. So, for example, while considering the suitability of DVT prophylaxis equipment for a particular patient, they will be reassessing the choice and how effective it is or might be while undertaking the task. This type of reflection is commonly associated with experienced practitioners and Greenwood (1993) suggests that it is usually triggered by an unexpected result or even surprise while the experience or activity is happening.

Schön's real contribution was revealing how professionals cope with complex problems and the type of reflection that supports this – either reflection on or in action – identifying limitations and guiding future development (Schön 1983: 68):

> The practitioner allows himself to experience surprise, puzzlement, or confusion in a situation which he finds uncertain or unique. He reflects on the phenomenon before him, and on the prior understandings which have been implicit in his behaviour. He carries out an experiment which serves to generate both a new understanding of the phenomenon and a change in the situation.

However, ODPs' experiences in perioperative care are usually time-critical – decisions need to be made and having time for reflection and consideration is unrealistic. But what is evident is that despite not closely following a 'textbook' theme, as practitioners, we do still think things through and, as every case is unique, we do have to draw on the experiences that have gone before to help us.

Reflecting on professional practice or undertaking reflection as an academic requirement in this way can help you to understand yourself as it may make your personal feelings, such as biases, expectations and beliefs, far more evident to you. Understanding yourself, in terms of your learning, knowledge and personal feelings, can support your studies and developing professional practice, as it will make you aware of potential assumptions that can be made almost automatically if you do not set out to reflect consciously on your actions or why you have done things a certain way.

Ways to reflect

Essentially, there are three ways to do this: as an individual, with another (such as a mentor, peer or colleague) or as a group. The experience and what you hope to gain (learn) from the process will usually determine which option you choose, but this may differ from occasion to occasion and you may use one or more ways for each experience.

Reflecting involves:

- thinking through an experience – reflection on practice;
- thinking back on an experience happening now – reflection in practice;
- reflective writing, such as reflective reports, accounts or essays, learning logs, activity logs, diaries or journals, critical analysis, email, social networks;
- reflecting with another – for example, talking through an experience with a peer or colleague, in a tutorial, clinical supervision, appraisal, presentation, email, social networks;
- group reflection in, for example, reflective group work, seminars or presentations, during or following role play or a simulation, a team debrief session or a critical incident analysis.

Reflecting on your own can be as simple as mulling over the experiences of the day on your way home or making entries in a diary or log of activities. Often this process will not develop beyond the descriptive, so opportunities to really 'unpick' the events or turn the thoughts into action or learning are not realized. Reflective writing is a strategy that can be used for many purposes and does allow for a more thoughtful and structured approach to emerge. While it is far more prevalent in those who are undertaking some formal learning at any stage of their development (whether as a pre-registration student or an advanced practitioner), it is undoubtedly a valuable way in which to become a 'consciously reflective practitioner' (Jasper 2003: 143). It also forms a record of your activity and learning that could be used as evidence, for example, in an assessment for a student (which will be considered later) or evidence of CPD if you are a practitioner or taking part in an HCPC audit. Alternatively, consider the case of an ODP who has undertaken a mentorship course. Mentorship, whether as initial preparation for a role or updating, is commonly an activity ODPs undertake as part of their professional development. To put this in the specific context of the HCPC's audit process, developing mentorship skills is counted as demonstrating CPD.

The first two standards relate to the 'experience' or 'What?' in Borton's (1970) model.

Standard 1: Maintain a continual, up-to-date and accurate record of their CPD activities
This will be a list of all your CPD activities (Section 5 of profile) during the audit period. *Your mentorship course must be on this list.*

Standard 2: Demonstrate that their CPD activities are a mixture of learning activities relevant to current or future practice
Your mentorship CPD could be a number of activities. For example, formal learning, if you attended a course; online workshop to update; student feedback on your performance as a mentor, reading, peer evaluation or appraisal. If you look back, your mentorship was probably a combination of these activities.

The next two standards relate to 'reflection' or 'So what?' and 'action' or 'Now what?' in Borton's (1970) model.

Standard 3: Seek to ensure that their CPD has contributed to the quality of their practice and service delivery
You need to discuss here how your mentorship CPD has made you (or was undertaken to make you) a better mentor. It may be that you are not yet a mentor but are planning to be, so a mentorship course, for example, may be part of the plan to achieve this goal. This may mean essential updating is undertaken, in terms of students' programme requirements, or you felt that better time management or giving feedback were areas you needed to develop.

Standard 4: Seek to ensure that their CPD benefits the service user
You need to identify your service users in the context of mentorship CPD. It is likely that these will be students, but the department, education manager or higher education institute (HEI) may also be considered.

Standards 3 and 4 are the most critical and in-depth part of your profile and form Section 3 of the HCPC's template. The aim of this part is to demonstrate how the CPD has been of benefit to you and others. It is the value of the activities that counts rather than what you have done – how the experience and what you have learnt have contributed to developing you. Therefore, the reflective process is fundamental to this being achieved.

Standard 5 encapsulates the whole framework, presenting the 'What?', 'So what?' and 'Now what?' in Borton's (1970) model in the context of the practitioner's role and development needs.

Standard 5: On request, present a written profile, which must be their own work and supported by evidence explaining how they have met the standards for CPD
From your list of CPD activities, select three or four samples to discuss in your profile, one of which could be your mentorship CPD. The authenticity of these will be assessed and evidence of the activities needs to be provided. For example, you could include a mentorship certificate of achievement, student feedback (anonymous), a critique of the literature, excerpt from an appraisal, peer evaluation or personal reflection.

Figure 5.2 Example of integrating the ERA framework with the HCPC's standards for CPD

Every two years, a number of ODPs are selected for a CPD audit. If selected, you will need to submit a profile (the HCPC will provide the template for this). The profile has five sections. Section 1 is simply your profession and unique CPD number. Section 2 is a brief summary of your current and aspirant role, as appropriate. Sections 1 and 2 therefore set the context. Section 3 is a personal statement, which evaluates your CPD in relation to standards 3 and 4 by using the three stages of the Experience, Reflection and Action (ERA) framework – 'experience' in this case being the mentorship course, and by 'reflecting' on this you will analyse how and why this has improved your practice and contributed to other service users. In your analysis, you will 'action' developments or opportunities for future practice and service delivery. The penultimate section, section 4, is the evidence submitted in support of the selected CPD being discussed and, finally, section 5 is the list of all your CPD for the period covered by the audit, both of these, therefore, providing the evidence that you have met the standards. The key to presenting your CPD to the HCPC when selected for audit, therefore, is to do so using a reflective process, conveying the value it has been to you. Figure 5.2 sets this in context by showing how the standards are met via such a reflective process.

Less formally, as part of your role as an ODP, you will be continually reflecting with others but, whether one to one or as a group, it does bring with it some challenges as well as advantages. The advantages include seeing things from another's perspective, using others as a sounding board for ideas, drawing on the expertise and experience of others, being asked questions that you may not ask yourself, finding alternative actions and bringing a new context or objectivity to the fore. It is vital also to be aware of the challenges involved in reflecting with others and the need to have clear ground rules in place at the outset, which should include strict adherence to standards of professional conduct (HCPC 2016) and an awareness of the consequences, such as issues with confidentiality, disclosure and emotional control.

Increasingly, reflecting with others takes place on social networking sites, such as Twitter, Facebook and Instagram, and any other communication media available that offer avenues for reflective practice with others. Reflective and dialogic learning are clearly identified in the e-learning pedagogy, the 'connectivist' learner being most likely to use a social network environment (Conole et al. 2010). Social networking is dominated by Facebook, which has more than 3.5 billion users – that is 45 per cent of the world's population (Statistic Brain Research Institute 2020). It is therefore appropriate to consider the use of social networking in relation to reflective strategies in this chapter.

Clearly, social networking media has revolutionized the way people connect socially. However, there are potential challenges, which bring this warning, that with such online activities, the professional integrity of registered practitioners, and those aspiring to be registered, could be called into question, as the blurring of personal and professional boundaries can easily occur. Even employing the strictest privacy settings, any information placed on a social networking site is considered to have been put in the public domain. There, it could be viewed by people other than those the originator may have intended, therefore having the potential to breach confidentiality. Social networking used appropriately can be an asset to your communication networks, but you can all too easily get caught up in a chain reaction of negative events that cross boundaries of professional and personal life.

Toolkit for reflection

A number of frameworks or models exist that will help ODP students and registrants to structure their reflection. The Williams report resulted in a recommendation to all healthcare regulators to clarify their position on the use of reflection. As a result the HCPC (2021) published guidance to support registrants, provided a toolkit and gave reassurance regarding how to use reflection in both CPD and fitness to practice cases (visit its website for a wealth of resources). Developing the skill of reflection will allow you to analyse and evaluate your learning experiences in greater depth, enabling you to progress your practice or be able to move on to more advanced study and learning.

Three models of reflection are described in this section, two of which are among the most commonly used and widely known models in healthcare (Jasper 2003; Wigens 2006) and the third offers an alternative view that may be more

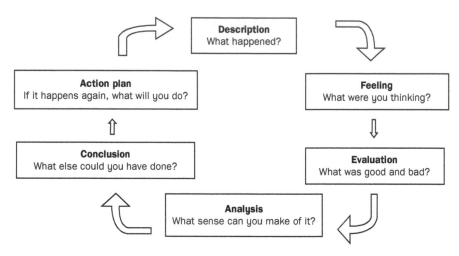

Figure 5.3 Reflective cycle

Source: Adapted from Gibbs (1988)

useful for reflecting in groups or with one other. First, Gibbs' six-stage reflective cycle is described (see Figure 5.3), followed by Borton's (1970) three-stage model (see Figure 5.4) and, finally, the model suggested by Dyke (1990: Figure 8.6).

Gibbs' reflective cycle

This model has six stages.

Stage 1: Description – what happened?

Describe in detail the event you are reflecting on. Include things such as where you were, who else was there, why you were there, what were you doing, what other people were doing, what the context of the event was, what happened, what your part in this was, what parts other people played and what the result was.

Stage 2: Feelings – what were you thinking?

At this stage, try to recall and explore those things that were going on inside your head. Include:

- how you were feeling when the event started;
- what you were thinking about at the time;
- how it made you feel;
- how other people made you feel;
- how you felt about the outcome of the event;
- what you think about it now.

Stage 3: Evaluation – what was good and bad about the experience?

Try to evaluate or make a judgement about what has happened. Consider what was good about the experience, what was bad about it or what did or did not go so well.

Stage 4: Analysis – what sense can you make of It?

Break the event down into its component parts so they can be explored separately. You may need to ask more detailed questions about the answers to the last stage. Include:

- what went well and why you think that was;
- what you did well;
- what others did well;
- what went wrong or did not turn out how it should have done;
- the way you or others contributed to this.

Stage 5: Conclusion – what else could you have done?

This differs from the evaluation stage because you have explored the experience from a number of angles, gaining further information on which to base your judgement. Remember, the purpose of reflection is to learn from an experience. Without detailed analysis and honest exploration in all the previous stages, it is unlikely that all aspects of the event will be taken into account and, therefore, valuable opportunities for learning can be missed. During this stage you should ask yourself what you could have done differently.

Stage 6: Action plan – If It happens again, what would I do?

During this stage you should think about planning what you would do next time – would you act differently or would you be likely to do the same? Do you need to get some training, gain new knowledge or learn about new equipment for example?

Here, the cycle has been notionally completed, but should the event occur again, it will be the focus of another reflective cycle, to continually develop your professional practice. Gibbs is closely aligned to Kolb's learning cycle and works on the premise that theory and practice continually enrich each other in a never-ending cycle.

Gibbs' reflective cycle has been widely adopted in healthcare as a way to facilitate reflection and it is a model that most ODPs are likely to be familiar with. However, while it does offer a basic and clear way to structure reflection, it is also criticized as needing to be developed into a broader and more critical reflexive approach (Jay and Johnson 2002).

Borton's model

Borton's (1970) model is very simple and is a good one for the novice reflector. It provides a starting point for student and registrant ODPs to first make sense of experiences and then respond to real situations.

It uses three key questions – 'What?', 'So what?' and 'Now what?' – which can be further supported with a number of cue questions for each, such as the following.

What?

- What happened?
- What did I do?

- What did others do?
- What was I trying to achieve?
- What was good or bad about the experience?

So what?

- So why did it happen?
- So what is the importance of this?
- So what more do I need to know about this?
- So what have I learnt about this?

Now what?

- Now what could I do next time?
- Now what else do I need to do?
- Now what might I do?
- Now what might be the consequences of this action?

Figure 5.4 provides a fictitious example of an ODP student using Borton's model following a first placement where they had to reflect on one experience to demonstrate how HCPC professional standards could be illustrated.

As you can see, this is a simple but effective way of formalizing a learning experience through reflection. Borton also tends to focus on reflection *on* action, looking back at an experience, rather than *in* action. A more experienced reflector may not opt for this model as a consequence. Emotions and feelings can be problematic and cause a novice reflector to get 'bogged down' in the initial stages, so this may be easier to start with than Gibbs' reflective cycle. Equally, however, the deeper understanding of these emotions is an important part of the reflective process that enables learning to take place. The key thing to come out of the process is for you to come to know yourself and understand how you learn best.

Dyke's framework for experiential learning and critical reflection

While Kolb's, Gibbs' and Borton's models are familiar to ODP students and qualified practitioners alike, and have been evaluated as useful learning tools, there is a concern that can limit the development of critical reflection. Hull et al. (2005) challenge Kolb and Gibbs, arguing that their models present a false picture and suggesting that they do not reflect the real world as it does not necessarily act so systematically and analyse each state on each occasion.

Joyce (2011) found that student ODPs frequently reflected together and, more widely, perioperative practitioners engage in team briefings and debriefings on a regular basis, as part of the World Health Organization's 'WHO guidelines for safe surgery 2009' (WHO 2009), so it seems a weakness of encouraging the use of models such as the two described previously in this section is that they promote individual reflection, which fails to engage ODPs in a more social way for collective reflection. Indeed, this was the argument of Guille and Young (1998), who suggested that the social context is a key part of reflection in reflexive learning. 'Reflexivity' and 'reflexive' are words used frequently in connection with professional and personal development. Reynolds (1998) suggests four characteristics that clearly distinguish critical reflection from reflection:

Reflection on foundation placement

Introduction

I am a first-year student Operating Department Practitioner (ODP) reflecting on the experience of my first placement, the foundation placement. Reflection is identified as a key way in which we can learn from experiences undertaken (Jasper 2003). I will be using Borton's framework of reflection (Jasper 2003), which provides a simple, logical structure so I can focus on my learning and development, and allows for a greater understanding of the experience (Ghaye 2005).

I will use the three prompt questions from Borton's model – 'What?', 'So what?' and 'Now what?' (Jasper 2003). My reflection will incorporate the use of evidence to support practice and make reference to professional standards where appropriate.

What?

The placement was a four-week introductory phase of my clinical experience, during which time I had eight outcomes to achieve that focused on communication and health and safety areas. These were all achieved and I have selected one specific experience to reflect on. In my third week I went with my mentor to do a preoperative visit to a patient due in theatre later that day. The patient was sitting by her bed, chatting to her husband. My mentor introduced herself and allowed me to do the same, at which point she tactfully interjected and took over the conversation.

So what?

When I introduced myself to the patient, I explained that I was a student and would also be present during her surgery. At the time, I had started to say the actual operation, which is when my mentor carefully took over the conversation. After the visit, my mentor explained that unless consent has been given to discuss any aspect of personal information or surgery in front of family or relatives, it is a breach of confidentiality (Health and Care Professions Council (HCPC) 2023). The HCPC's Standards of conduct, performance and ethics (2016) also highlight the need for every patient to be dealt with individually and respectfully, always acting in the patient's best interests. The intervention from my mentor ensured the patient was not compromised in any way, but also protected me from breaching confidentiality, which I had not realized it was so easy to do.

Now what?

Evaluating this event has increased my awareness of patient confidentiality, consent, data protection and identifying situations where this can so easily be breached, and not to make assumptions about what a close relative may or may not know. If a similar situation arises again, I will be able to make an informed decision about gaining consent or considering options to ensure that I maintain confidentiality (HCPC 2023).

Conclusion

I have reflected on one event from my foundation placement. The structured process of a framework such as Borton's (Jasper 2003) has allowed me to analyse the situation constructively and consider the professional issues in relation to this. I have recognized the development needs arising from this, which is an essential skill for an accountable practitioner.

References

Ghaye, T. (2005) *Developing the Reflective Healthcare Team*. Oxford: Blackwell.
Health and Care Professions Council (HCPC) (2016) Standards of conduct, performance and ethics. London: HCPC.
Health and Care Professions Council (HCPC) (2023) Standards of proficiency: Operating Department Practitioners. London: HCPC.
Jasper, M. (2003) *Beginning Reflective Practice*. Cheltenham: Nelson Thornas.

Figure 5.4 Example of student using Borton's model in a structured reflection

- question assumptions;
- social not individual focus;
- analysis of relations;
- emancipation.

So, when ODPs reflect critically, they do far more than just look back on or reflect in an experience and unpick the events; they also look at the wider environment in which they are situated. This allows them to consider the social stance and even power or influences exercised by the organization, through its networks and wider relationships. While, often, they cannot impose transformational change or action at organizational level, this does encourage ODPs to not be inhibited by such barriers to change as, for example, 'that is the way things are done here' culture.

Dyke (2009) offers an alternative framework for experiential learning, one that is far more flexible than those discussed so far in this section. As with other frameworks or models, ODPs are still encouraged to include the theory, what they know; how this is applied, the experience itself; and reflect on these to inform future practice, but Dyke's model (2009: 306) does not rely on sequential steps or conforming to any direction. There are no arrows and so no order of events, which serves to support developing students to learn more effectively and, importantly, recognizes the need to reflect with others.

Learning is often reliant on an experiential approach and reflection is a vehicle for this. But we need to consider whether the strategy used is restrictive in much the same way as, in clinical practice, when a number of clinical algorithms are applied that are to be followed religiously, so offering a model of reflection means that it will probably be adhered to in the same way. Figure 5.5 is adapted from Dyke's original model, which demonstrated a lack of order and conformity, without the straight and regimented lines to follow that can be found in the more traditional frameworks described earlier in this section. If the signposts that suggest direction and sequence were removed as Dyke suggests, then the process would become more fluid, more critical and potentially of greater benefit to both ODPs and students as they reflect with others in a team. My adaptation of this model (see Figure 5.5) shows the four aspects randomly connected, but maybe of differing importance (indicated by size), with the central tenet being the opportunity to *reflect with others*. This is imperative for ODPs, as teamwork is such an important player in perioperative practice.

Stop and think

Consider an experience in the past week in your professional practice.

What would be different if you consciously reflected as a perioperative team rather than individually?

Some of the issues you may have considered will be those already discussed as the consequences of reflection. But the nature of your relationship in any group

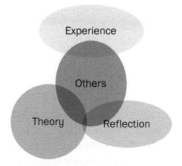

Figure 5.5 Dyke's framework for reflexive learning

Source: Adapted from Dyke (2009)

may change and the structure of a group is likely not to be rigid so may result in a deeper and broader analysis of an event than would be achieved by reflecting on it alone. The importance of what happens here will be the effect on and actions of the team as a whole and the professional development of that team.

Conclusion

Hopefully this chapter has provided you with an overview of reflection from the perspective of an ODP. While there is little empirical evidence that reflection can improve patient care (Mann et al. 2009), it has been proven to enhance the process of care, as it is associated with a deeper approach to learning, allowing it to be integrated with existing knowledge and skills. There is no mystique attached to the process of reflection. In its simplest form, it is a process of learning from experience, whether it is the passive decision-making concerning day-to-day activities such as eating or doing the washing, or the extremes of critical thinking and transforming the very culture of the organization that we are in.

Reflection is not without consequences and challenges to ODPs. It may well trigger emotional responses that will need to be dealt with, find challenges in the relationships with colleagues, highlight biases and assumptions and even issues of confidentiality and professionalism if undertaken in the public domain of social networking or without forethought.

We have seen that a range of models is available to guide practitioners though the structured process of reflection, of which four have been considered in this chapter. Different models may be needed for every experience and which one is chosen can be influenced by the event itself, the individual and the context of their role at the time. The development of professional practice will benefit from this type of diversity, however, and it is important to apply models purposefully, selectively and judiciously.

Key points

- Reflection is a key aspect of development, education and re-registration for ODPs.
- Reflective practice can be defined as a process to make sense of experiences, events and actions in the practice environment.
- It is a valuable process for enhancing professional practice, improving effectiveness and advancing lifelong learning as an ODP.
- Reflective practice is not without its challenges and consequences.
- It enables ODPs to manage their learning and development.
- A toolkit of models to support and guide reflective practice is available to be used appropriately by ODPs.
- Effective reflection can be conducted as an individual, with another, in teams or groups or a mix.
- Reflection should not be ritualistic or limited by an algorithmic approach to applying a model or ticking boxes.
- Reflection can allow more critical levels of thinking to emerge and develop.

References and further reading

Borton, T. (1970) *Reach, Touch and Teach*. London: Hutchinson.

Boud, D., Keogh, R. and Walker, D. (1985) *Reflection: Turning Experience into Learning*. London: Kogan Page.

College of Operating Department Practitioners (CODP) (2018) Bachelor of Science (Hons) in Operating Department Practice – England, Northern Ireland and Wales; Bachelor of Science in Operating Department Practice – Scotland: Curriculum document. London: CODP.

Conole, G., Brown, R., Papaefthimiou, M., et al. (2010) Fostering connectivity and reflection as strategic investment for change, in U.D. Ehlers and D. Schneckenberg (eds), *Changing Cultures in Higher Education*. New York: Springer.

Dewey, J. (1933) *How We Think: A Restatement of the Relation of Reflective Thinking to the Educative Process*. Chicago, IL: Henry Regnery Co.

Dyke, M. (2009) An enabling framework for reflexive learning: Experiential learning and reflexivity in contemporary modernity, *International Journal of Lifelong Education*, 28(3): 289–310.

Eraut, M. (1994) *Developing Professional Knowledge and Competence*. Abingdon: Routledge Falmer.

Finlay, L. (2008) Reflecting on 'reflective practice'. Discussion paper 52. Buckingham: Open University.

Fitzgerald, M. (1994) Theories of reflection for learning, in A. Palmer and S. Burns (eds), *Reflective Practice in Nursing*. Oxford: Blackwell Scientific.

Gibbs, G. (1988) *Learning by Doing: A Guide to Teaching and Learning Methods*. Oxford: Oxford Polytechnic.

Greenwood, J. (1993) Reflective practice: A critique of the work of Argyris and Schön, *Journal of Advanced Nursing*, 19: 1183–7.

Guille, D. and Young, M. (1998) Apprenticeship as a conceptual basis for a social theory of learning, *Journal of Vocational Education and Training*, 50(2): 173.

Hargreaves, J. (2004) So how do you feel about that?: Assessing reflective practice, *Nurse Education Today*, 24(3): 196–201.

Health and Care Professions Council (HCPC) (2016) Standards of conduct, performance and ethics. London: HCPC.

Health and Care Professions Council (HCPC) (2017) Standards of continuing professional development. London: HCPC.

Health and Care Professions Council (HCPC) (2019) Benefits of becoming a reflective practitioner: A joint statement of support from Chief Executives of statutory regulators of health and care professionals. London: HCPC.

Health and Care Professions Council (HCPC) (2021) Reflective practice: Recognise, reflect, resolve: The benefits of reflecting on your practice. London: HCPC.

Health and Care Professions Council (HCPC) (2023) Standards of proficiency: Operating Department Practitioners. London: HCPC.

Hobbs, V. (2007) Faking it or hating it: Can reflective practice be forced?, *Reflective Practice*, 8(3): 405–17.

Hull, C., Redfern, L. and Shuttleworth, A. (2005) *Profiles and Portfolios: A Guide for Health and Social Care*, 2nd edn. New York: Palgrave.

Jasper, M. (1999) Nurses' perceptions of the value of written reflection, *Nurse Education Today*, 19(6): 452–63.

Jasper, M. (2003) *Beginning Reflective Practice*. Cheltenham: Nelson Thornes.

Jay, J.K. and Johnson, K.L. (2002) Capturing complexity: A typology of reflective practice for teacher education, *Teaching and Teacher Education*, 18, 73–85.

Johns, C. (1995) A philosophical basis for nursing practice, in C. Johns (ed.), *The Burford NDU Model: Caring in Practice*. Oxford: Blackwell Scientific.

Joyce, P. (2011) Professional confidence in Diploma of Higher Education Operating Department Practice students. Published thesis, University of Southampton.

Kolb, D. (1984) *Experiential Learning as the Science of Learning and Development*. Upper Saddle River, NJ: Prentice Hall.

Mann, K., Gordon, J. and Macleod, A. (2009) Reflection and reflective practice in health professions education: A systematic review, *Advanced Health Science Education*, 2: 1573–677.

Reynolds, M. (1998) Reflection and critical reflection in management learning, *Management Learning*, 29(2): 183–200.

Sandars, J. (2009) The use of reflection in medical education: AMEE Guide no 4, *Medical Teacher*, 31: 685–95.

Schön, D. (1983) *The Reflective Practitioner*. New York: Basic Books.

Smyth, J. (1992) Teachers' work and the politics of reflection, *American Educational Research Journal*, 29(2): 267–300.

Statistic Brain Research Institute (2020) Social networking statistics. Global: Statistic Brain Institute. Available at: www.statisticbrain.com/social-networking-statistics (accessed September 2022).

Wigens, L. (2006) *Expanding Nursing and Health Care Practice*. Cheltenham: Nelson Thornes.

Williams, N. (2018) Gross negligence manslaughter in healthcare: The report of a rapid policy review. Review commissioned by Jeremy Hunt, Secretary of State for Health, UK government. Available at: https://assets.publishing.service.gov.uk/government/uploads/system/uploads/attachment_data/file/717946/Williams_Report.pdf (accessed September 2022).

World Health Organization (WHO) (2009) WHO guidelines for safe surgery 2009: Safe surgery saves lives. Geneva: WHO. Available at: www.who.int/teams/integrated-health-services/patient-safety/research/safe-surgery (accessed September 2022).

6 Patient safety and Operating Department Practitioners

Keith Underwood and William Kilvington

Key topics

- Human factors:
  - the dirty dozen
  - situation awareness with a case study
  - devices, ergonomics and training
  - tall man lettering and administering drugs safely
- WHO guidelines for safe surgery and the five steps for safer surgery
- The 'Never Events' framework:
  - National Safety Standards for Invasive Procedures (NatSSIPs)
- Root cause analysis (RCA)
- Other safety models:
  - Reason's Swiss cheese model
  - Reason's three bucket model
  - iceberg theory
- Safeguarding issues:
  - vulnerable adults
  - children
  - learning disabilities

Introduction

In this chapter, we introduce key aspects relating to patient safety. There is no one, standalone text that encompasses the whole subject of patient safety so, to ensure that you have an appropriate level of knowledge when caring for patients, it is necessary to gain an understanding of the basic principles of the subjects concerned. The principles as set out in this chapter are an initial guide to what you need to know to underpin your practice. This must then be supplemented by further reading to increase your understanding as the principles apply to each *specific* area of your practice.

In every section, we have therefore provided some key words or phrases to search for when you research the principles further.

Much of the learning that we apply to safety in healthcare has come from other industries in which safety is also critical, such as aviation and nuclear energy. In particular, what we now understand as the 'human factors' in patient safety were largely developed from learning in aviation following a series of catastrophic accidents in the 1970s and 1980s. The introduction of flight data and cockpit voice recorder technology, so-called 'black boxes', gave unprecedented insight into human behaviour and inputs as contributory factors to air accidents. Significantly, mechanical failure alone rarely leads to serious air accidents.

Although black box technology has yet to be widely adopted in healthcare, its value in simulations for assessing team dynamics and performance is now recognized.

Why is this relevant?

Concerns about patient safety are probably as old as medicine itself and the doctrine 'Primum non nocere', which means to 'first, do no harm', is widely attributed, if erroneously, to Hippocrates ($c.460$BCE–$c.375$BCE). Modern clinical practice has introduced levels of complexity undreamed of even early on in the working lives of some current Operating Department Practitioners (ODPs) and, while technology has done much to improve care and safety, such complexity brings its own hazards. The weakest link in the safety chain still remains the 'human factor'.

As with general health and safety at work principles, patient safety in perioperative care is the responsibility of all, not only the manager. Indeed, it is the responsibility of each individual practitioner, irrespective of grade or title. For multidisciplinary team members to work effectively to provide optimum care, we must understand hazards, the risks they give rise to and how these risks are mitigated or militated against.

While it is right for clinical staff to focus on the human cost and impact of clinical errors, the economic impact should not be ignored. The NHS Resolution 'Annual report and accounts 2019/20' (2020) shows that the annual cost of harm arising from clinical activity was £8.4 billion, and the provision for all unmet claims was set at £84.1 billion. In comparison, the NHS England budget to commission services in the same period was £121 billion.

Human factors

You cannot change the human condition, but you can change the conditions in which humans work

(Reason and Hobbs 2003)

Human factors in healthcare – sometimes known as 'non-technical skills' – have been defined as:

enhancing clinical performance through an understanding of the effects of teamwork, tasks, equipment, workspace, culture and organisation on human behaviour and abilities and application of that knowledge in clinical settings.

(Catchpole et al. 2010)

Human behaviour is complex and, in 1993, Gordon Dupont developed the concept of the so-called 'dirty dozen' factors (Aviation Knowledge 2010) while working for Transport Canada, which are:

- lack of communication
- distraction
- lack of resources
- stress
- complacency

- lack of teamwork
- pressure
- lack of awareness
- lack of knowledge
- fatigue
- lack of assertiveness
- norms (developed culture – 'the way we do things around here').

It is not difficult to see how each of these factors is directly applicable to our roles in perioperative care, although it can be more challenging to mitigate against them in teams. We can, of course, take personal responsibility for our own knowledge, well-being and behaviour, but inadequate resources, pressure and the behaviour of others are seemingly out of our control.

That is when assertiveness becomes important and, in healthy teams, every member is empowered to speak up when they are concerned about an aspect of care. A key part of being a healthcare professional is having the 'professional courage' to speak out at such times. A key aspect of being a leader is creating an environment of 'psychological safety' that empowers such courage.

'Situational or situation awareness' can be defined as the perception of environmental elements and events in relation to time or space, the comprehension of their meaning and projecting what their future status will be. Loss of situation awareness is a common factor in adverse events, especially in dynamic, complex situations where information overload can overwhelm the senses. Conversely, familiarity with a task and complacency can also lead to an inappropriate response or action.

Stop and think

Situation awareness has three key elements. Read the descriptions of these elements in the following list and think of situations in which you may be able to apply these.

- **Perception** – how the individual 'sees' things. This varies from individual to individual and in a given situation. Loss of situation awareness is a frequent contributing factor to adverse incidents. An individual can become so focused on something specific that they miss or block out other important information and cues.
- **Comprehension** – understanding what you are seeing or being told. A classic example in healthcare is focusing on a machine alarm, thinking it is a fault, rather than on what is really happening with the patient.
- **Projection** – considering what may happen in the near future given the information that is available now.

Can you think of examples when intense focus during a surgical procedure could lead to a clinician losing situational awareness and how you, as the ODP, might intervene?

Search for: 'human factors dirty dozen', 'human factors in healthcare', 'professional courage in healthcare', 'situation awareness in healthcare'

The power gradient, personalities and staff interaction

Personalities in any team, but especially a multidisciplinary team, easily create communication barriers. In a perioperative team, you could have senior and experienced medical, nursing and ODP members of staff, who have significant levels of competence and the confidence to say how they feel about any given situation. This might also be a team of people who are used to working together and understands each other's idiosyncrasies, so will probably work well in both the routine and stressful situations. It is not uncommon for members of staff who work closely together and have clinical experience to be able to anticipate each other's needs. An anaesthetic practitioner who gets the atropine just before the anaesthetist asks for it, and a scrub practitioner who places the correct instrument into the surgeon's hand without any verbal indication as to what they require are signs of experience and teamwork. However, such moments can be experienced between individuals who have not worked together in a team before or between one inexperienced individual and others when they are working in a recognized team. Either way, the team dynamics and communication in these situations will be different from those in an established team. This is simply a result of being human as, while we like to work with people we know, there may be situations when we seek explicit guidance or leadership and/or we need to take the lead role.

The 'power gradient' observable in an operating theatre has existed as long as operating theatres themselves. There is a perceived ladder of the ranks of the professionals who work together in the perioperative environment, and different roles may be considered to be at different levels within those ranks. However, for a team to work as effectively as possible, this power gradient needs to be flattened.

In any team, when managing a critical situation, there needs to be a leader who the other members of the team look to for instructions. In an operating theatre, there might, in fact, be two at any one time, such as the anaesthetist and the surgeon, but what needs to be remembered is that no individual can see and hear everything when they are concentrating on completing complex practical tasks in a stressful situation. It is therefore of paramount importance that all members of the team are empowered to say what they think, when they think it should be said. This is how the power gradient can be flattened.

When thinking about vocalizing a concern in a given situation, the use of a graded approach to assertiveness can be useful for those who are less comfortable about raising an issue. This can be used as a tool to escalate concerns. Phrases that could be used to do this could be, to start, 'I have some concerns', then on to, 'I really don't understand' and, finally, 'I think we should stop, as I feel that there is a safety issue'.

Senior members of staff or those with authority have a responsibility to listen to others and create an environment that is psychologically safe for any member of the team to raise a concern, and they should 'gift' them the ability to speak up if needed.

It is important to recognize that professional courage may be required to speak out assertively when a situation demands it.

Search for: 'power gradient in healthcare', 'psychological safety at work'

Stop and think

When looking at how well teams work together and other aspects of team dynamics, there will always be a difference between an acute and a routine situation. Think about some examples from your practice and why these differences occur.

The ergonomics of devices and training

Human factors also influence the design and use of medical devices, a process commonly known as 'ergonomics'. The configuration of buttons, for example, can make a difference to how they are used. Modern medical devices for administering drugs and fluids – such as syringe drivers and volumetric infusion pumps – when produced by the same company, may have similar, if not identical, layouts for buttons and screens. Doing this not only helps with training in their use but can also help when members of staff are dealing with critical incidents. For this reason, hospitals and departments seek to standardize their equipment.

One change that has been incorporated in some newer devices is that the entering of numbers for the required dose and/or volume has been replaced with up and down arrows or chevrons, a dial-up system or equivalent. This change has been made to reflect how we use such equipment. With a number pad, there is an increased potential for the wrong amounts to be entered, as individuals tend to pay more attention to the buttons they are pressing than to what is on the screen.

In a hospital environment, particularly in critical care, the numbers of medical devices we come into contact with can be quite significant, and they are potentially complex to use. The introduction of new devices into a department, therefore, must be managed well and appropriate training given. Remember, 'use' may well be defined differently depending on who you are and who you are asking. A couple of aspects that should be looked at for all devices, to ensure that they are used correctly, are appropriate training packages and whether these should be competence based, plus user manuals, instructions for use (IFU) and quick reference guides (QRG). User manuals, IFU and QRG, whether printed or in a digital format, need to be readily available to staff in the clinical areas in which the devices are used.

Stop and think

Think about the last new medical device that was introduced to your clinical area. Did you receive appropriate training? Was it competency based? Did you feel both competent and confident in its use after training or would you have benefited from anything having been done differently?

Search for: 'medical device ergonomics', 'MHRA medical device training'

'Tall man lettering'

Another area that is potentially problematic is that of misreading drug information (Underwood 2012). According to the Medical Protection Society (MPS 2012), the National Patient Safety Agency (NPSA, which became NHS Improvement after 2012 and then part of NHS England in 2022) had operated a National Reporting and Learning Service (NRLS) that received about 5,000 reports a month about patient safety incidents related to medication.

'Tall man lettering' was introduced in the pharmaceutical industry around 2008 to help improve the situation by making it easier for people to differentiate between 'look alike' and 'sound alike' (LASA) drug names. This form of labelling later became required for generic cephalosporins by NHS Improvement and the Medicines and Healthcare Products Regulatory Agency (MHPRA 2020). You will find that tall man lettering is becoming more frequently used by the pharmaceutical industry and being incorporated in not only both syringe drivers and volumetric infusion devices as part of their device drug libraries but also on the electronic pharmacy lists for wards and departments, and the labelling of the drug boxes themselves. As an example, as part of a procurement of the CareFusion Alaris GH+ syringe driver, 30 pre-programmed drug names were added to the device. Some of the drug protocols included in those pre-programmed drug names are AMINOphylline, AMIODARone, DOBUTamine, DOPamine, doPEXamine, FUROSemide and NORadrenaline. This short list shows how the names are given on the packaging and appear in the devices when using tall man lettering. If you see drug names in this unusual form, you will know that it probably is not a misprint but might be using tall man lettering, which has been done to help you identify a drug correctly, making the administering of that drug safer for the patient. You might also see the use of different colours for the text on drug packaging and this, too, is part of the tall man lettering system.

Stop and think

Have you come across tall man lettering where you work? If so, do others you work with understand why this format is in used?

Search for: 'tall man lettering'

The WHO guidelines for safe surgery and the five steps for safer surgery

The World Health Organization's (WHO) 'WHO guidelines for safe surgery' (WHO 2009) is a 19-step tool that has been shown to reduce complications and mortality associated with surgery by more than 30 per cent. Since its introduction the guidelines have been modified to suit local circumstances or particular specialties or procedures. Since 2010 the three stages in the WHO's guidelines have been incorporated into the following five steps for safer surgery, which should now have been adopted throughout the UK.

1 **Briefing** before commencing the surgical list or individual patient (if the team changes for each patient). Should be completed with all members of the perioperative team present. During the team briefing, each member of staff and their roles are introduced. List order and any concerns in relation to equipment, staff, anaesthesia, surgery should be raised. For example, regarding patients' positions on the list, should a patient be first or last due to latex allergies or MRSA or COVID status? Discussing these and other pertinent issues at the outset enhances safety and efficiency.

2 **Sign-in** takes place before the induction of anaesthesia. This confirms the patient, procedure and consent details. Concerns about allergies, airway issues, anticipated blood loss or special medications are discussed at this point and machines and medicines are checked.

3 **Time out** is when the team stops for a moment before starting surgery. Team member introductions are repeated and there is a final confirmation of the patient information and surgical procedure that is to take place. Also, the availability of the surgical site infection bundle and thromboprophylaxis imaging are confirmed.

4 **Sign out** occurs before any staff leave the theatre. There is confirmation of the recording of the procedure and that all swabs, instruments and sharps are accounted for. A check is done that specimens are correctly labelled and any equipment issues are addressed. Post-operative management is discussed and handed over.

5 **Debriefing** is completed at the end of the list or a procedure as part of the evaluation. This is an opportunity to learn from incidents and remedy problems, such as equipment failure, and to agree responsibilities for any actions arising. The evaluation should include positive aspects of the session, what went well.

In certain acute circumstances, it may be impractical to complete the safe surgery guidelines and five steps for safer surgery as intended. In these circumstances they should be looked on as tools to be used as effectively as possible. The WHO has acknowledged this and as part of its information package also discusses the situation for an emergency patient.

Search for: 'five steps for safer surgery', 'WHO safe surgery checklist'

The Never Events framework

In 2009 the concept of 'Never Events' was introduced in the NHS in England and since that time the Never Events policy and framework has been updated on a regular basis.

The policy and framework define 'Never Events' as 'Serious incidents that are wholly preventable because guidance or safety recommendations that provide strong systemic protective barriers are available at a national level and should have been implemented by all healthcare providers' (NHS Improvement 2018).

The list of Never Events categorizes them under four headings: surgical, medication events, mental health and general healthcare. The surgical Never Events comprise three types of events: wrong site surgery, wrong implant or prosthesis and retained foreign object post-operation. The list of specific events is under continual review and items may be added to the list as protective barriers become more robust. Conversely, specific procedures may be removed from the list, when it is deemed that the barriers are inadequate. For example, in 2021, the review removed wrong tooth extraction from the list because of ongoing issues with agreed nomenclature of teeth, including differences between adult permanent teeth and deciduous teeth in children. Although no longer a Never Event, this would still be classified as a serious incident (SI) and investigated as such.

Stop and think

The use of the term 'Never Event' remains contentious in some circles, principally because, despite the name, these events continue to happen. The provisional full-year data from 1 April 2020 to 31 March 2021 (NHS England and NHS Improvement 2021) shows that the following numbers of surgical Never Events were reported:

- wrong site surgery, 142
- wrong implant or prosthesis, 30
- retained foreign object, 80.

Using the definition of Never Events given earlier in this chapter, consider the measures in place regarding the events in this list and why they still have happened.

Search for: 'Never Events framework', 'Never Events statistics'

National Safety Standards for Invasive Procedures (NatSSIPs)

In 2013, the Secretary of State for Health (England) called for a Surgical Never Events Taskforce to be formed and its report, 'Standardise, educate, harmonise: Commissioning the conditions for safer surgery' (NHS England Patient Safety Domain 2014), led to the creation of a set of National Safety Standards for Invasive Procedures (NatSSIPs) in 2015. These were then implemented in England and Wales.

In January 2023, the NatSSIPs 2 were published by the Centre for Perioperative Care (CPOC) and these are a progression of the original standards, involving collaboration across the four nations of the UK and the significant learning that arose from this process. The NatSSIPs 2 represent a return to the aims of the original Surgical Never Events Taskforce's report, to standardize, educate and harmonize.

The NatSSIPs 2 are arranged in two interrelated sets of standards: the organizational and the sequential standards. The organizational standards set out the expectations of the roles of trusts and external bodies, which are to support teams to provide safe invasive care. The sequential standards expand the five steps for safer surgery to become the 'NatSSIPs 8' – that is, the eight steps to be taken, where appropriate, by individuals and teams for every patient having an invasive procedure.

Organizational standards	Sequential standards
1 People for safety	Consent and procedural verification
2 Processes for safety	Team briefing
3 Performance for safety	Sign-in
4	Time out
5	Implant use
6	Reconciliation of items
7	Sign out
8	Debriefing or handover

The Surgical Never Events Taskforce's report contains patient vignettes that illustrate the impacts of errors on patients.

Search for: 'NatSSIPs', 'Surgical Never Events Taskforce'

Root cause analysis (RCA)

NHS England (2015), in its 'Serious incident framework', has defined serious incidents (SIs) as 'adverse events, where the consequences to patients, families and carers, staff or organisations are so significant or the potential for learning is so great, that a heightened level of response is justified'. Following an SI, a common approach to an investigation is to complete a root cause analysis (RCA).

There are numerous sources of information regarding RCAs, but the key point to remember is that it is not important which system is used; what is important is how well it is used. You will get better results using a simple system well than you will by using a complex system badly. Taking this approach is not only important for establishing underlying causes and learning from them but also because the results of any investigation must be shared with the patient or their relatives. This 'duty of candour' is enshrined in law, in Regulation 20 of the Health and Social Care Act 2008 (Regulated Activities) Regulations 2014.

In the RCA we look at later in this chapter (see Box 6.3), there are six key factors that need to be considered. These are measurements, materials, personnel, environment, methods and machines. By using a process as simple as a fishbone, or, Ishikawa diagram, starting an RCA is straightforward. Terms commonly used in such an event review analysis are 'adverse incident', 'significant event', 'serious incident', 'serious untoward incident', 'near miss' and 'Never Event'. The key NHS-specific definitions of these terms are shown in Box 6.1 to help give you a better understanding of the terminology.

Box 6.1 Definitions of terms commonly used in root cause or event review analysis

- **Serious incident:** A situation in which one or more patients or staff are involved in an event that would present a significant danger to patients, visitors or staff, or is likely to generate significant legal, media or other interest that, if not properly managed, may result in loss of the trust's reputation, services or assets.
- **Near miss:** An unplanned event that had the potential to cause damage, injury or illness, but on this particular occasion did not.
- **Never Events:** Serious incidents that are wholly preventable because guidance or safety recommendations that provide strong systemic protective barriers are available at a national level and should have been implemented by all healthcare providers in those situations.

The seriousness of an incident should also be taken into consideration, remembering that in any incident it may not include 'damage' to a patient or staff member. The seriousness could be defined as given in Box 6.2.

Box 6.2 Categories used to classify the seriousness of an incident

- **Major:** This could include penetrating injury, loss of life, causing unconsciousness, loss of sight and the need for additional and/or prolonged treatment.
- **Moderate:** This could include drug administration errors with no lasting effects, verbal or physical abuse or fraud.
- **Minor:** This could include minor theft, slips, trips and falls resulting in little injury and vandalism.

Note: These lists are for illustrative purposes only and are not exhaustive.

An RCA, then, is a process for looking at all aspects associated with a given situation, analysing any potential and/or actual problems or incidents and developing a plan to ensure that, wherever practicable, it will not happen again. These situations could be related to a critical incident, serious event, near miss or a recognized Never Event. As a process, an RCA can be conducted at a departmental, trust, regional, national or even international level and need not be negative. For example, an international RCA was completed some years ago and the results have significantly altered the way we all work in operating departments. The outcome of that RCA was the 'WHO guidelines for safe surgery' initiative (WHO 2009).

The overall process of conducting an RCA is not new to healthcare management or operating theatres. In the past, we looked at issues or situations that had occurred, discussed problems and came up with plans to ensure they did not happen again. As technology and techniques have progressed, this approach led to the process we have now, which needs to be reviewed and documented accurately and, where needed, incidents reported appropriately, to the trust, the relevant regional authority or, potentially, at the national level.

Part of the process is to develop an appropriate action plan, which will often need to be linked to the trust's risk and legal department and the patient safety team. This overall process will probably start with an online reporting system, such as the Datix adverse incident reporting system (AIRS), but there are others. Which system is used in your clinical area is not important, but what is important is that it is used appropriately, correctly, accurately and in a timely manner.

If, in Box 6.3, we now consider the six factors mentioned previously – measurements, materials, personnel, environment, methods and machines – and expand them using general operating department terminology, we can see how this RCA framework can work for ODPs and provide information about an 'incident'.

Box 6.3 Example of the kinds of factors to take into account when the RCA framework is applied to a perioperative environment

- **Measurements:** Calibration of instruments and devices, dosages (mg, mcg, ml, mm, for example), printouts from devices and information stored on devices.
- **Materials:** Cleaning agents, suppliers, latex in products, control of substances hazardous to health (COSHH) data sheets and availability.
- **Personnel:** The time of day (such as shift patterns), staffing numbers, appropriate training, mixes of skills, who was there, whether students or other learners were present and the availability of senior staff.
- **Environment:** Time of day, temperature, humidity, lighting and where the incident occurred.
- **Methods:** Local and national policies, procedures, standard operating procedures, national standards and/or requirements.
- **Machines:** The devices used, servicing records, whether training was appropriate, the correct devices were chosen for the purposes they were used for, software was up to date, device protocols were signed off appropriately, checklists completed, brackets and attachments were used.

There are two points to remember:

1 The factors given in the RCA framework do not form an exhaustive list – they are intended as a basis for you to use to go on and develop your own thought processes.
2 Depending on the incident, not all the factors will be relevant, so do not try to find something for each factor – if you do, that is OK; if you don't, then that is fine too.

An RCA in practice

To understand the RCA process further, let us explore using it for an incident that did not result in a long-lasting injury to a patient.

While sliding Mr D (anaesthetized) from the bed to the operating table, he fell between the two and landed on the floor. So what are the things we need to look at and consider? By using the six factors of the RCA framework, hopefully it will give us all the information we require.

- **Measurements:** There is probably nothing of relevance to this case to mention for this factor.
- **Materials:** It will be necessary to examine the brake systems for the bed and table – were the brakes applied?
- **Personnel:** For this factor, we would look at the members of staff involved, their individual experiences, training requirements and training status (is their training up to date?). Remember that training requirements and training status are very different. For the training we would be looking at current competence regarding moving, handling and using medical devices for all the members of staff who were involved, irrespective of grade or profession. We could also consider the time of the day as this could have two influences, on the number of members of staff available and the level of fatigue they might be experiencing due to shift patterns.
- **Environment:** For this factor, we should consider where this occurred. Was it a suitable place to perform this move and would the time of day have played a role?
- **Method:** This is probably the most important issue to look at, along with the training of the individuals involved. We would need to consider if there are any standard operating procedures for the task in hand – moving the patient – what those procedures prescribe and if there is evidence that the individuals involved were aware of them. It is not uncommon for standard operating procedures (SOP) to be placed in a departmental folder with a read and sign sheet. If this had been done in this case, then the signature sheets would need to be examined and would form part of the overall evidence.
- **Machines:** Again, for this section it would be necessary to look at the training requirements regarding the medical devices used and to see if there were any faults affecting the wheel-locking mechanism for the bed and/or the table. This would give us some idea as to whether they items could both be locked in place before moving the patient. It would be imperative that the devices' asset numbers or serial numbers were recorded on any incident form and/or notes, so that the appropriate tests could be made as part of the RCA.

We should also be aware that each member of staff involved could well be required to complete a report on the incident that detailed what they did and said prior to and at the time of the incident, to gain a full picture of what happened.

From this you will see how looking at individual case studies is a good way to get a better understanding of the RCA process. To this end, try using it to look at an event you experienced in the 'Stop and think box'.

Stop and think

Think about a case you have been in involved in where an aspect did not go to plan. Reflect on this using the RCA framework.

Multiskilled practitioners

Having multiskilled practitioners in perioperative care is an advantage, benefiting both clinical functioning and patient care. Some recognized multiskilled roles are:

- anaesthetics and PACU
- anaesthetics and surgery
- PACU and surgery
- surgery, anaesthetics and PACU
- anaesthetics and/or PACU + trauma and/or resuscitation and/or inter-hospital transfer teams.

Such practitioners can fulfil many roles, not only in the operating department but also in other areas and in specialist teams. There is a view that the multiskilled practitioners in a department can enhance patient safety because, it is perceived, they have a better understanding of the patients' journey through the department. We should also acknowledge, however, that this would not be the effect in all areas, with all staff and not all the time. Therefore, having 'specialist' practitioners that cover individual areas should also be considered and not viewed negatively by other practitioners or management when developing team dynamics. The aim should always be to be patient centred and all issues concerning communication and the 'WHO guidelines for safe surgery' (WHO 2009) adhered to, ensuring patients' safety.

Stop and think

What do you do if the surgical list you are working through alters? For example, what if the order changes, making Mrs J, who was third on the list, fifth. Has this information been communicated appropriately to all relevant parties in and outside the theatre complex? What alterations need to be made in the department to accommodate this change? Does this happen where you work and, if so, how is it managed?

Search for: 'anaesthetic and surgical practitioner', 'safe theatre practitioner', 'theatre practitioner NHS'

Recognized safety models frequently applied to healthcare

Reason's Swiss cheese model

In 1990, James Reason propounded the Swiss cheese model as a tool for risk analysis and management. The model – introducing multiple layers of defence to avoid any single points of failure leading to a harm event – has been widely adopted in healthcare.

Reason's model is so called as it is based on slices of Swiss cheese, placed in a line. Each slice represents a system barrier to a harm event. The model propounds that any barrier is likely to have flaws or holes, like those in Swiss cheese. The implication is that where one barrier fails, then the next in the chain is effective and prevents harm. A serious harm event is likely to occur only when the holes in the barriers align.

Earlier in this chapter we discussed the five steps for safer surgery training and the deployment of new equipment. Each is an example of a layer of Swiss cheese.

Search for: 'Swiss cheese effect in healthcare'

Stop and think

Can you describe how each of the five steps for safer surgery build on one another to strengthen barriers so as to avoidable patient harm?

Reason's three bucket model

Another of Reason's (2000) methodologies is a tool to provide foresight when assessing risky situations. The three buckets are labelled 'self', 'context' and 'task'. By placing 'bad things' in each of the buckets, you can assess the level of risk presented under each category by how 'full' your buckets are.

The bad things represent inadequacies or gaps assessed under each heading:

Self	Context	Task
Level of knowledge	Equipment and devices	Errors
Level of skill	Physical environment	Task's complexity
Level of expertise	Workspace	Novel task (rare, new, unfamiliar)
Current capacity to do task	Team and support Organization and management	Process

By identifying the bad things, it is possible to develop strategies for mitigating the risks in each area. There are various three bucket templates available online that you can try.

Search for: 'three bucket model'

Stop and think

Consider a situation when you thought that a clinical activity had not gone as well as you expected or wished. Using the three buckets model, try to 'load' the three buckets with what could have been contributory factors to this situation.

The iceberg theory

This theory has been applied across a wide range of sectors and contexts and is often applied to organizational culture and safety. The simple premise is based on the fact that only 10 per cent of an iceberg is visible above the waterline. In terms of culture and safety, similarly, what you see is only the tip of the iceberg, and what is going on below the waterline is what matters.

In the context of safety, serious incidents are the tip of the iceberg and near misses are an indication of what is going on below the waterline. If we focus on reducing or eliminating the near misses, the tip of the iceberg – the serious incidents – will also be reduced.

Search for: 'iceberg model healthcare safety'

Stop and think

Ask your organization or department's safety team to provide you with a report of the two most recent serious incidents and five near misses reported.

Using the information provided, consider if there are any common themes that could be indicative of factors that underlie them both.

Safeguarding – key elements of patient safety

So far in this chapter we have considered specific aspects related to patient safety, but it is important to note that safeguarding is a fundamental part of caring for patients that may extend beyond the clinical aspects of your role.

Ensuring that patients are cared for safely is not only dependent on the systems, processes and having an understanding of the aspects of human behaviour discussed previously in this chapter. It also requires careful consideration being extended to those who have particular needs or vulnerabilities.

'Safeguarding' is defined by NHS England (n.d.) as 'protecting a citizen's health, wellbeing and human rights, enabling them to live free from harm, abuse and neglect'. This definition provides a comprehensive statement that can be used to guide practices in your specific legislative framework. Further, each nation in the United Kingdom has its own legislation for safeguarding vulnerable groups (see the 'Further reading' section at the end of this chapter for links to learn about their provisions and some guidance), some of which are:

England
The Care Act 2014
The Children Act 1989 (as amended)

Scotland
Adult Support and Protection (Scotland) Act 2007
Children and Young People (Scotland) Act 2014
Getting it right for every child (GIRFEC)

Wales
Social Services and Well-being (Wales) Act 2014
Wales Safeguarding Procedures

Northern Ireland
Safeguarding Board Act (Northern Ireland) 201

Those most in need of safeguarding include children and young people, as well as adults at risk. This can include those with sensory, physical or mental impairments or a learning disability. Safeguarding vulnerable individuals in a healthcare setting is the responsibility of all staff, clinical and non-clinical, so it is important to be aware of the six principles that underpin safeguarding in practice in all health and care settings, which are:

* **empowerment:** People need to be supported and encouraged to make their own decisions and be enabled to give informed consent;
* **protection:** Support and representation need to be in place for those in greatest need;
* **prevention:** It is better to take action before harm occurs;
* **partnership:** Find local solutions through services working with their communities, and communities have a part to play, too, in preventing, detecting and reporting neglect and abuse;
* **proportionality:** Make the least intrusive response appropriate to the risk presented;
* **accountability:** There needs to be accountability and transparency in safeguarding practice.

Safeguarding training in most healthcare organizations forms part of the package of statutory and mandatory training that is required for all staff. The level and frequency of training is dependent on the individual's role and level of contact with vulnerable individuals or groups.

Vulnerable adults and children

It is important to understand the essential terminology used (such as 'vulnerable adult', 'abuse' and 'abuser'). Each organization will have definitions that it uses for these terms and, although the meanings will be the same, the wording could well vary slightly from one organization or part of the country to another, so it is important that you know your own organization's definitions. See Box 6.4 for some examples.

Box 6.4 Terminology used in relation to vulnerable adults and children

Term	Meaning
Vulnerable adult	An individual over the age of 18 and, for some reason, unable to look after themselves. This might be because of physical or mental health problems, age, illness or learning disabilities
Abuse	Where one or more people say or do something that causes physical, mental, emotional or sexual harm to an individual. It can also be where an individual's civil or human rights are violated
Abuser	Any individual can be an abuser – friend, relative, carer or unknown to the individual

Adult-specific training

Training in organizations is usually broken down into set levels relating to individual members of staff or practitioner grades. The Association of Directors of Social Services' (2005: 20) national framework of standards for good practice for protecting vulnerable adults (summarized in Box 6.5) is an example of how training for members of staff may be organized.

Box 6.5 Example of good practice for structuring training for members of staff in protecting vulnerable adults

As a minimum, ODPs should achieve Level 1, which is having an understanding of what might constitute abuse and what actions they should take when they witness or suspect abuse.

Course outline

Level 1
Awareness: Developing a shared understanding of what abuse and what a vulnerable adult is and an understanding of the signs and symptoms of abuse. Also, what to do if you witness abuse or are told about it.

Level 2
The practitioner's role: How to deal with disclosures for those who need to complete the alert form as part of their professional role. How to determine risk, vulnerability and seriousness.

Examining the implications of the three 'Cs' – capacity, consent and confidentiality.

Level 3
The investigator's guide: The knowledge and skills required when planning and undertaking a protective and/or detective (collecting information) investigation, either as a single agency or jointly with colleagues from other agencies. Examining elements of good practice when gathering evidence.

Level 4
Joint working and criminal investigations: Developing mutual understanding of the complementary and supportive roles of the police, social services and other agencies when a potential crime has been committed. This will include an overview of the 'achieving best evidence' model of interviewing.

Level 5
Decision-making: This course is directed at those who will be involved in the conclusive decision-making processes (such as care conferences and planning meetings) and have responsibility for these under the current policy and procedures. Also included will be evaluating the evidence and implementing protection planning.

Level 6
Post-abuse: Establish who the stakeholders are regarding protection planning. How to provide for the post-abuse support needs of the vulnerable adult and their support networks – a strengths and needs model. How to manage the impact of adult protection on practitioners.

(Association of Directors of Social Services 2005: 20)

It is generally considered that all staff working in the NHS should understand how to safeguard vulnerable adults, irrespective of their own role, whether it is clinical or non-clinical. The level of training will need to be increased if you are expected to recognize signs of abuse, are accountable for responding to these or for investigating issues concerning safeguarding alerts.

Child-specific training

The Royal College of Nursing's publication, 'Safeguarding children and young people', otherwise known as the 'Intercollegiate document' (RCN 2019), is a key document covering this area of training. It provides a framework and describes the training requirements for safeguarding this age group, which are set out as five levels of competence (see Box 6.6).

Box 6.6 Training requirements relating to safeguarding children and young people

Target audiences for the course

Level 1
All members of staff working in healthcare services.

Level 2
All non-clinical and clinical members of staff who have contact (however small) with children and young people and/or parents/carers or adults who may pose a risk to children.

Level 3
All clinical members of staff who work with children, young people and/or their parents/carers or any adults who could pose a risk to children and those members of staff who could potentially contribute to assessing, planning, intervening and/or evaluating the needs of a child or young person and/or parenting capacity (regardless of whether there have been previously identified child protection/safeguarding concerns).

Level 4

For those with specialist roles, such as named professionals working in safeguarding children and young people.

Level 5

For those with specialist roles, such as those designated professionals working in safeguarding children and young people.

(RCN 2019)

It is important that ODPs understand their personal responsibilities and training needs, and how the impact this has on their professional accountability. ODPs should be aware of what training is required and should make sure that they keep up to date with both general and departmental issues at all times. ODPs working with children should access the higher levels of training.

Stop and think

You are providing care for a three-month-old child and notice bruising around their lower limbs and back. You remember a phrase used during your safeguarding training, 'If they're not cruising, they're not bruising'.

What do you think this means and what is the appropriate action that you should take in this situation?

Learning disabilities

ODPs should consider what impact they have on the experience of patients with a learning disability (LD) in a perioperative environment. The Department of Health (DH), in its 'Six lives' progress report (2013), looks specifically at 'what has happened to make things better for people with learning disabilities since the Department of Health's "Six Lives" progress report in October 2010'.

Stop and think

Imagine you have been seconded to provide care for a patient in a high-dependency escalation area. The patient you have been asked to care for is a 40-year-old woman with a serious chest infection. The patient also has trisomy 21, otherwise known as Down's syndrome.

In reviewing the health record, you note that the patient has a 'do not attempt resuscitation' order (DNAR/DNACPR) in the file.

Now think about the safeguarding implications of this information and what action, if any, you should take.

Conclusion

This chapter has highlighted some of the key themes concerning safety in perioperative care and why and how we should use systematic approaches, such as the five steps for safer surgery. The fallibility of the human condition has been a focus, along with techniques and understandings aimed at minimizing any adverse impacts associated with our very human condition.

We have explored the duties and responsibilities of ODPs to the most vulnerable in our care. We are used to working in those stages of perioperative care where a service user's voice cannot be heard, but in this chapter we have stressed the importance of paying attention to the voice of the vulnerable in our care and those whose capacity to understand and consent is diminished.

Throughout this chapter we hope that we have maintained a focus on the most important aspect of this subject: keeping our service users safe. Although we have used the terms 'patient' and 'patient safety' earlier, here we have reflected the language most commonly used by the Health and Care Professions Council (HCPC), which is 'service user', as this should help us to frame our relationship appropriately with those under our care.

Finally, we see all too frequently headlines about failures in care and how healthcare providers do not learn the lessons arising from those failings. One of the reasons for this is that we do not read the reports so do not pick up on the lessons they offer us. Thus, our final search terms have been chosen to point you in the direction of some of those key reports and the learning that can be gleaned from them. We have also included terms that will take you to patients' stories and the impacts their experiences have had on them and their families. Many of these make for uncomfortable reading, but hopefully it will help to motivate you to be a better, safer practitioner.

Search for: 'Berwick review', 'Francis report 2013', 'Morecambe Bay investigation', 'action against medical accidents', 'harmedpatientsalliance.org.uk', 'patientstories.org.uk', 'patientvoices.org.uk'

Key points

- Patient safety in the operating department is a key responsibility of all members of a multidisciplinary team, irrespective of job title or role. Therefore, patient safety should be considered a 'team game' at all times.
- When completing any RCA, greater emphasis should be placed on completing the process correctly than on the complexity of the system you are using.
- All members of staff should be aware of the appropriate policies in relation to safeguarding vulnerable adults and children.
- Members of staff should understand their employer's stance on LD, know what provisions are in place generally and those available in their own work area.
- It is advisable that individuals are conversant with NHS Improvement's 'Revised Never Events policy and framework' (2018), which includes the updated Never Events list, remembering that these are fluid, so should be reviewed regularly.

References and further reading

Association of Directors of Social Services (2005) Safeguarding adults: A national framework of standards for good practice and outcomes in adult protection work. London: Association of Directors of Social Services.

Aviation Knowledge (2010) The 'dirty dozen' in aviation maintenance. Aviation Knowledge. Available at: http://aviationknowledge.wikidot.com/aviation:dirty-dozen (accessed November 2022).

Catchpole, K.R., Dale, T.J., Hirst, D.G., et al. (2010) A multicenter trial of aviation-style training for surgical teams, *Journal of Patient Safety*, 6(3): 180–6.

Centre for Perioperative Care (CPOC) (2023) National Safety Standards for Invasive Procedures 2 (NatSSIPs 2). London: CPOC.

Department of Health (DH) (2013) Six lives: Progress report on healthcare for people with learning disabilities. London: DH.

Medical Protection Society (MPS) (2012) Medication errors. London and Leeds: MPS Available at: www.medicalprotection.org/ireland/booklets/avoiding-problems-managing-the-risks-in-general-practice-in-ireland/medication-errors (accessed 17 November 2022).

Medicines and Healthcare Products Regulatory Agency (MHPRA) (2020) Best practice guidance on the labelling and packaging of medicines. London: MHPRA. Available at: https://assets.publishing.service.gov.uk/government/uploads/system/uploads/attachment_data/file/946705/Best_practice_guidance_labelling_and_packaging_of_medicines.pdf (accessed November 2022).

NHS England (n.d.) About NHS England safeguarding. London: NHS England. Available at: www.england.nhs.uk/safeguarding/about (accessed July 2023).

NHS England (2015) Serious incident framework: Supporting learning to prevent recurrence. London: NHS England. Available at: www.england.nhs.uk/wp-content/uploads/2020/08/serious-incidnt-framwrk.pdf (accessed November 2022).

NHS England and NHS Improvement (2021) Provisional publication of Never Events reported as occurring between 01 April 202 and 31 March 2021. London: NHS England. Available at: www.england.nhs.uk/wp-content/uploads/2021/05/Provisional-publication-NE-1-April-2020-31-March-2021.pdf (accessed November 2022).

NHS England Patient Safety Domain (2014) Standardise, educate, harmonise: Commissioning the conditions for safer surgery. Report of the NHS England Never Events Taskforce. London: NHS England. Available at: www.england.nhs.uk/wp-content/uploads/2014/02/sur-nev-ev-tf-rep.pdf (accessed November 2022).

NHS Improvement (2018) Revised Never Events policy and framework. London: NHS Improvement. Available at: www.england.nhs.uk/patient-safety/revised-never-events-policy-and-framework (accessed November 2022).

NHS Resolution (2020) Annual report and accounts 2019/20. London: Her Majesty's Stationery Office.

Reason, J. (1990) The contribution of latent human failures to the breakdown of complex systems, *Philosophical Transactions of the Royal Society London B, Biological Sciences*, 327(1241): 475–84.

Reason, J. (2000) Human error: Models and management, *British Medical Journal* (Clinical Research Edition), 320: 768–70.

Reason, J. and Hobbs, A. (2003) *Managing Maintenance Errors: A Practical Guide*. Farnham: Ashgate Publishing.

Royal College of Nursing (RCN) (2019) Safeguarding children and young people: Roles and competencies for healthcare staff, Fourth edition: Intercollegiate document. London: RCN.

Available at: www.rcn.org.uk/Professional-Development/publications/pub-007366 (accessed November 2022).

Underwood, K. (2012) Are you short or TALL?: Reducing risk of drug errors, *Technic*, 3(3): 6–7. Archived by the College of Operating Department Practitioners (CODP).

World Health Organization (WHO) (2009) WHO guidelines for safe surgery 2009: Safe surgery saves lives. Geneva: WHO. Available at: www.who.int/teams/integrated-health-services/patient-safety/research/safe-surgery (accessed November 2022).

Further reading

Anderson-Wallace, M. (2013) *Beth's story* (film, 15 minutes). Patient Stories. Available at: www.patientstories.org.uk/films/beths-story (accessed August 2023).

Clinical Human Factors Group. Available at: https://chfg.org (accessed October 2022).

Donaldson, L., Ricciardi, W., Sheridan, S., et al. (2021) *Textbook of Patient Safety and Clinical Risk Management*. Cham, Switzerland: Springer.

Empowered Patient (2013) Hospital guide for patients and families. The Empowered Patient Coalition. Available at: www.engagedpatients.org/empowered-patient-hospital-guide-patients-families (accessed November 2022).

NHS England (2019) Access the following link for a set of webpages as further reading regarding enduring standards that remain valid from previous patient safety alerts up to November 2019. Available at: *www.england.nhs.uk/patient-safety/patient-safety-alerts/enduring-standards/standards-that-remain-valid/surgical-anaesthetic-maternity-safety* (accessed November 2022).

Reason, J. and Hobbs, A. (2003) *Managing Maintenance Error: A Practical Guide*. Farnham: Ashgate Publishing.

Safe Surgery 2020 (n.d.) Safe Surgery 2020: Impact report. Safe Surgery 2020. Available at: www.safesurgery2020.org (accessed November 2022).

Legislation

England

The Care Act 2014: www.legislation.gov.uk/ukpga/2014/23/contents/enacted (accessed November 2022).

The Children Act 1989 (as amended): www.legislation.gov.uk/ukpga/1989/41/contents (accessed November 2022).

Scotland

Adult Support and Protection (Scotland) Act 2007: www.legislation.gov.uk/asp/2007/10/contents (accessed November 2022).

Children and Young People (Scotland) Act 2014: www.legislation.gov.uk/asp/2014/8/contents/enacted (accessed November 2022).

Getting it right for every child (GIRFEC): www.gov.scot/policies/girfec (accessed November 2022).

Wales

Social Services and Well-being (Wales) Act 2014: www.legislation.gov.uk/anaw/2014/4/contents (accessed November 2022).

Wales Safeguarding Procedures: www.safeguarding.wales (accessed November 2022).

Northern Ireland

Safeguarding Board Act (Northern Ireland) 2011: www.legislation.gov.uk/nia/2011/7/notes#:~:-text=The%20Act%20will%20provide%20the,area%2C%20to%20support%20the%20SBNI (accessed November 2022).

Safeguarding Board for Northern Ireland Procedures Manual: www.proceduresonline.com/sbni (accessed November 2022).

7 | Psychosocial aspects of operating department practice

Christine Mahoney and Daniel Rodger

Key topics

- Clarification of terms
- Redefining care in health settings
- Psychosocial theories and their importance for perioperative practice

- The balance of power and control
- Psychosocial changes across the lifespan
- Stigma and the group mentality

Introduction

This chapter introduces some of the theories behind people's behaviour and offers Operating Department Practitioners (ODPs) a basis on which to consider their current practice when supporting and caring for perioperative patients.

There are several definitions of 'psychology', but it is generally considered to be the study of thought and behaviour, the object of which is understanding why people behave as they do. 'Sociology', however, is the study of human social behaviour, focusing particularly on the organization and development of human society. Sociology looks at the ways humans interact with one another rather than focusing specifically on the sense of self. The combination of psychology and sociology gives rise to the phenomenon of the 'psychosocial', which includes the nature of people's own behaviour, and how that behaviour may affect or be affected by interaction with others.

Why is this relevant?

Everything that ODPs do requires interaction with other humans, often under heightened emotional conditions and within a specific timeframe, with the associated pressures those factors bring. In stressful work environments it is easy to become task-orientated, which can mean that patients feel (at best) *attended to* rather than *cared for*. Equally, staff-to-staff communication may become less effective when under stress, which may cause the team's performance to be compromised. Indeed, failure in communication is the most common cause of errors and adverse events in operating theatres (Etherington et al. 2019). Gaining a deeper understanding of the underpinning tenets of human behaviour enables practitioners to appreciate what makes each person an individual, to consider current practice and find ways to enhance interactions with all those in the theatre environment.

Redefining care in health settings

There has been a tremendous growth in recent years of policies (both in the UK and internationally) aimed at improving the 'care' of patients. These have largely emerged in response to high-profile cases reported in the media where failures in a system have led to inadequate care in various sectors of health and social care. Two such high-profile failures are what occurred at the Mid Staffordshire NHS Foundation Trust between 2005 and 2009, resulting in the Francis inquiry, and the Maternity Services at the Shrewsbury and Telford Hospital NHS Trust between 2000 and 2019, the subject of the first Ockenden report (2020). The first Ockenden report reviewed the care of 250 mothers and their babies; the final report (2022) explored the cases of nearly 1,500 families. At the core of every government-led inquiry into such failures is an individual human being who has suffered at the hands of those from whom they expected a satisfactory level of care and, in the process, that human being has become a statistic.

In an effort to re-establish the human context of the numerous reports, policies and protocols, it may help to reconsider what is meant by 'care' in a health setting and, in particular, in the perioperative environment.

The *Cambridge Dictionary* (2021) defines care as, 'the provision of what is necessary for the health, welfare, maintenance, and protection of someone or something'. This, of course, could be achieved in a mechanistic, task-orientated fashion, but patients deserve more than such a basic level of attention. There has been growing dissatisfaction with the medical model, which is when patients are viewed as passive recipients of care and treatment is focused on correcting the relevant medical symptom in the patient's body. In contrast, it is now recognized that 'care' should encompass much more than this – it should be more holistic and patient-centred. It needs to involve showing empathy, considering the patient's spiritual needs, respecting each patient as an individual, understanding their wishes and ensuring that they share in making decisions about their own care (Arakelian et al. 2017; Chen et al. 2017).

This psychosocial approach recognizes the ways in which human experience, culture and society influence our attitudes to health. The World Health Organization (WHO 1946) has defined health as 'a state of complete physical, mental and social well-being and not merely the absence of disease' and, although this view of health has been challenged by a change in the pattern of disease during the half century or so that has passed since it was written, mental and social well-being is still a central ideal in healthcare. People experience the National Health Service (NHS) at times of basic human need, when care and compassion are what matter most (Department of Health and Social Care (DH) 2012). Patients feel that shortfalls in care, impersonal treatment and lack of compassion reveal a lack of respect on the part of those practitioners who treated them in this way.

In a busy operating theatre department, the care of patients has many components, which will be delivered by several multidisciplinary staff. ODPs must communicate clearly, ensure safe patient positioning, check equipment, maintain infection control, act as an advocate for patients and ensure the accurate recording of events, which all contribute to the care of surgical patients (Rodger and Mahoney 2017). However, if the individual receiving such care does not feel that the ODP is compassionate, an opportunity to improve the patient's experience has been lost.

Stop and think

Consider the department you work in. Have you ever observed an individual receiving impersonal or off-hand treatment? Might this have happened when a patient is behaving 'differently' or is 'not communicating'?

Psychological theories and their importance for perioperative practice

Psychology, broadly speaking, is an attempt to explain why people behave as they do. Why does behaviour vary significantly between individuals faced with the same situation or, for that matter, why might a person behave differently in different circumstances?

What is a 'psychological theory'?

Psychologists have, over many years, developed several 'approaches' to the subject, and for each of these approaches (or perspectives) there are many individual theories. In each case, the theorist presents an argument for why a person may exhibit particular behaviour. Some theories are widely accepted, others hotly contested, and there is no conclusive evidence for any one of the specific approaches. Indeed, trying to analyse an individual's behaviour from only one psychological perspective would be impossible – humans are far too complex for that.

This broad range of explanations may lead you to deduce that none of the theories are accurate as they cannot be proved or disproved. From a purely scientific perspective, nothing is ever proved, and all findings remain theories until such times as further evidence can challenge their accuracy. From the psychologist's viewpoint, the theories provide a position that can be debated and discussed in relation to observable human phenomena.

It is difficult to imagine now that there was a time when these subjects were not the topic of debate, a time when no one considered it necessary to analyse behaviour or offer explanations for it. The various studies of the mind, and subsequent development of theories, have given people the vocabulary and a framework to talk about and understand human behaviour in a way that is now taken for granted. Thoughts or feelings may be described as 'subconscious' or 'unconscious', with a sound expectation that others will know what these terms mean. A person may be described as having a 'complex', and people will understand how that affects behaviour, yet these words were unheard of in this context until the latter part of the nineteenth century.

We will now consider several psychological approaches in relation to observable behaviour in an operating department. The intention behind this is to encourage you to broaden and increase your understanding of the basic psychological processes that you may see in the perioperative environment. The principal focus is on the impact of these on the perioperative care of patients but, of course, psychological theories can be applied to ODPs, too, and to team communication. Practitioners are encouraged to think of all aspects of their team roles when applying psychological and psychosocial theories to their practice.

The psychodynamic approach to psychology and the Freudian perspective

The 'psychodynamic approach' is a term used to refer to several theories that consider what drives or motivates humans to behave as they do and, in particular, the effects of the unconscious mind on behaviour. Sigmund Freud (1856–1939) remains the most influential psychodynamic theorist. Freud's psychoanalytic theory relies on the observation that human behaviour has its roots in early childhood experiences – often ones that we are unable to remember consciously. Perhaps most famously Freud postulated that the unconscious mind has three main parts – the 'id', 'ego' and 'superego'. Tensions between these three parts can cause anxiety, so people develop coping or defence mechanisms, which can be observed.

The 'id' is associated with basic, primal, innate instincts, principally to do with survival. According to Bruce and Borg (2002), Freud originally coined the term 'lib-id-o', meaning 'vital energy', but it has since come to be associated solely with sexual instincts. Freud's explanation of the id includes sexual instincts, but also covers aggression associated with self-protection, and he proposed that the id is incapable of logical thought.

The 'superego' responds to the morals and rules of society – what some people refer to as the mind's conscience. This part of the mind is thought to develop between the ages of about three to six years and it is what governs the ways we 'ought' to behave in society. The superego's role is to contain the desires of the id by observing the rules of society, and this can create tensions.

To apply these terms to your work as an ODP, a surgical patient's self-preserving id will want to run away from the terrifying experience of allowing strangers to undertake procedures from which the body may not recover. Their superego will be forcing them to 'behave nicely' in this situation because the staff are there to help and it is not acceptable to make a fuss. These competing reactions can start a cycle of mutually reinforcing events, such as aggressive self-protection and embarrassment at their inappropriate behaviour. This then serves to increase the patient's anxiety, as they may be feeling self-conscious already due to several other factors, including nudity, fear of the unknown and possibly a needle or other phobias.

The third of Freud's proposed parts of the mind, the 'ego', attempts to mediate between the id and the superego to find a balance. It does this by storing up previously experienced responses to specific stimuli and producing a response that is appropriate for dealing with a specific tension. The ego recognizes the tensions between innate, self-preservation instincts and the need to conform to society's rules, and employs a number of defence or coping mechanisms to fulfil its role as mediator. Examples of these coping strategies are clearly observable in perioperative patients, so ODPs need to know about, identify and respond to them. Here are some of the strategies you may come across.

- **Denial:** A patient may be unable to engage in discussion about the procedure or associated interventions. ODPs need to be aware of the signs of this, such as an inability to maintain eye contact or a focus on repetitive actions (such as folding and unfolding a tissue or plucking at the sheet on the bed).
- **Displacement:** This may manifest as becoming angry with others not necessarily involved in the immediate process. For example, blaming the ward staff for not explaining things properly or decrying the actions of whoever the patient may see as responsible for their being in hospital (the government, workplace or cat that they fell over).
- **Regression:** A patient may exhibit this by retreating to childhood behaviours that are seen as comforting, such as sucking their thumb or rocking back and forth with their arms wrapped around their knees.
- **Reaction formation:** This strategy involves replacing a type of behaviour that normally would be considered signs of weakness or inappropriate – crying, for example – with its opposite, such as overconfidence or being exceptionally chatty.

Stop and think

Freud's theories can be applied to staff as well as patients. Can you think of examples where a colleague's behaviour may be explained by the psychoanalytic approach? What might be provoking the id, and what might the ego be initiating to mediate their behaviour?

Freud's theories have been challenged by many as being too reductionist, trying to predict behaviour of all people based on the close examination of a few individuals. The abstract nature of his concept of self has also been questioned, but as the behaviours he described are evidently exhibited in people under stress, the approach may be seen as relevant and worthy of being believed by healthcare practitioners.

The behaviourist approach – reinforcement and conditioning

Another well-known psychological approach is 'behaviourism', founded by John B. Watson (1878–1958) in 1913 and later expanded by B.F. Skinner (1904–90), which has its roots in Pavlovian response theory. In direct contrast to Freud's introspective approach (looking at internal, abstract phenomena), behaviourists concerned themselves with observable reactions to specific external stimuli, and this approach dominated psychology for the first half of the twentieth century. Watson believed that personality develops because of learnt behaviours, which are mostly influenced by other people and the environment. As such, he suggested that objective scientific studies on stimulus and response could be undertaken, which would allow predictions to be made about behaviour in defined circumstances.

The behaviourist approach discounts internal personal motivation and focuses instead on stimulus–response interactions, which have come to be known as 'conditioning'. Ivan Pavlov's famous experiment that demonstrated dogs salivating whenever the idea of food was presented to them – not only once they actually saw the food – led to further studies on conditioned responses.

Conditioning happens because specific responses are repeatedly experienced in association with the same stimuli, so are expected. These associations can be positive or negative. A positive example may be a person who is inclined to undertake a particular process because a previous experience or experiences suggest that the outcome will be pleasurable. Perhaps due to scepticism, positive conditioning tends to be less evident than negative conditioning, which is when scenarios may be avoided because in the past they have caused pain or stress.

Upton (2012) describes a phenomenon known as anticipatory nausea and vomiting (ANV), which occurs among patients undergoing chemotherapy for cancer and is when they report nausea and/or vomiting prior to the chemotherapy drugs being administered. Such is the power of classical conditioning, that patients begin to feel nauseous on entering the ward or even when they attend the same hospital for another reason.

Negative reinforcement seems to be harder to challenge than positive reinforcement, and even if the stimulus does not produce the expected response, it takes a long while for the learnt behaviour to subside. For example, a person may develop a needle phobia after only one unpleasant experience. Any subsequent painless injections or cannulations would be viewed as exceptions or 'flukes' and so would not change the anticipatory behaviour of fear and withdrawal. Of course, fear initiates the stress response and so contributes to a negative experience, which is why a negative association cycle is particularly difficult to break.

Stop and think

How might hospital-induced anxiety be explained according to conditioning theory? Is there anything you could do as an ODP to alleviate the stress linked with an experience in the perioperative environment?

Related to conditioning is the concept of 'operant conditioning', whereby the individual has a role to play in influencing the outcome. That is to say, by exhibiting particular behaviours, a positive response (or reward) may be elicited.

Clearly, a real change in behaviour requires repeated exposure to the stimulus–reward concept. This may not be practicable in operating theatres as the patient interactions are too infrequent for the conditioned response to become established, but having an understanding of how this process works enables ODPs to appreciate how their behaviour may have an influence on their patients' future experiences. If, due to staff shortages or the pressures of a busy operating list, a practitioner fails to take time to give a patient their undivided attention, the patient's sense of being a nuisance or a bother will be reinforced. This might mean that, in future, that patient fails to divulge something of importance when questioned. Conversely, putting a patient at the centre of the therapeutic relationship will enhance feelings of trust and importance, which could make them less fearful of future experiences.

The expectation that a particular behaviour may elicit the same response in the future, because of past experience, is a learning theory proposed by Albert Bandura (1925–2021), one that is based on the behaviourist approach. Bandura (1977) proposed that people with a low level of expectancy (of reward) will put little effort into changing their behaviour. This low expectancy is often influenced by subjective observations of the behaviour of others, as well as past experiences of one's own perceived ability to change ('I can't lose weight no matter how I try – my mother was just the same,' for example).

This can be seen in what we call 'vicariously learnt' attitudes, such as children learning by observing their parents' or carers' behaviour. If a child sees that their mother or father is anxious about a visit to hospital, and that such a visit results in pain for the parent, then the child will be anxious that the same will happen to them if they go to hospital. This phenomenon is not unique to children; a response may become further reinforced over the course of someone's lifespan, resulting in adults who are still anxious or fearful based on the behaviour of their parents decades before.

Stop and think

How much of your professional behaviour is influenced by 'vicariously' learnt attitudes from your peers? Do you find yourself changing your behaviour depending on who you are working with? Do you ever find yourself using this as an excuse for your own behaviour?

The behaviourist approach went on to evolve into 'cognitive psychology', which focuses on the mechanistic processing of thought, based on the impersonal, logic-based flow diagrams now familiar to computer programmers. Much of the research into cognitive psychology relies on scientific, laboratory-based experiments and, as such, attracts the criticism that real life is not like a laboratory. The lack of a personal, emotional element in the various theories proposed by behaviourists encouraged a break away from this perspective and towards an approach that puts the human condition at the centre of psychological studies.

The humanist approach and the influence of identity

The 'humanist', or 'person-centred', approach developed as a reaction to the previous dominant themes in psychology. Based on the work of Abraham Maslow (1908–70) and Carl Rogers (1902–87), humanist theories focus on the emotional and physical needs of the human condition, and the concept of 'self'. The personal nature of human experience including love, creativity, hope, health, individuality and value are all viewed as components that add to the complexity of human behaviour. Both Maslow (1970) and Rogers (1951) firmly believed that people have a natural tendency to move towards health, growth and a positive self-concept, assuming the right conditions are present.

Maslow developed a model demonstrating how people will tend to move towards emotional and cognitive fulfilment, providing their basic 'life needs' are met. In simple terms, deficiency in any of the basic elements of human need (food, shelter, safety, love, respect) will prevent a person from achieving their full potential or 'self-actualization'. The human psyche, one might say, is concerned with self-preservation and recognition of its own value above any other less vital concerns, such as intelligence or beauty. When the whole human condition is under threat – during illness, for example – then, often, the lower-level needs (food, sleep and attention) take complete precedence and the higher-level concerns, such as personal attractiveness, are ignored.

Rogers agreed with Maslow but concluded that a person could not achieve this personal growth alone as they needed positive reinforcement from those around them in the form of genuineness, acceptance and empathy. He also made it clear that each person is unique – we each have their own 'pinnacle' of achievement, which will not be the same for anyone else, even someone who has encountered exactly the same environmental and emotional conditions. The sense of 'self' or identity – what makes each of us exactly who we are – is central to Rogers' theory of person-centred psychology.

In healthcare terms, this means that, to care effectively for an individual, ODPs need to take time to determine what it is that a person needs, not to make assumptions based on what would make them, the practitioners, feel better in the same situation. How often has the phrase 'treat patients as you would wish to be treated' been passed on from practitioner to learner? In Rogers' terms this should be rephrased slightly to 'treat patients as *they* would wish to be treated'.

Rogers' concept of 'self' includes two separate identities: real self (the person as they really are) and ideal self (the person they would like to be). If these two entities are vastly different, the person would feel uncomfortable, experiencing low self-esteem and lacking in confidence. To balance the two entities, a person requires permission (or positive regard) from those around them, even if they behave in a 'less than ideal' fashion.

If an ODP were to apply this theory to their perioperative patient, the patient's perception of their real self (anxious, helpless, a nuisance, unable to deal with the situation) will likely be far removed from their ideal self (confident, grown up, in control), and this will manifest in what may be termed 'disordered' behaviour. This could certainly result in anxiety or possibly aggression, rudeness or even withdrawal. For the ODP to be able to support the patient, the patient must perceive that the ODP has a genuine interest in their welfare, rather than an 'adopted' or professional attitude. ODPs need to develop the skills to connect with patients in this way. Patients in the perioperative environment need acceptance, empathy and, above all, 'congruent' or genuine communication. This means that words are not enough – practitioners, by their body language and by giving patients personal attention, reinforce the therapeutic nature of their communication.

Stop and think

Think about a situation that you encountered in the perioperative environment recently in which someone's behaviour appeared bizarre or 'unacceptable'. In the light of your understanding of psychological approaches from reading this chapter, can you now offer explanations for why they behaved this way, and how the situation might have been handled better?

Psychosocial theories and their importance for perioperative practice

Psychological theories can help to explain the behaviour of individuals, but it is recognized that social factors, such as their environment, culture and peer pressure, can also have impacts on their behaviour. People do not live or behave in isolation – the context of a social setting in which they are functioning will affect their behaviour. Thus, the term 'psychosocial' came into being to describe theories that seek to explore and explain the influence of such external factors.

Psychosocial theories focus on the premise that the human character is fundamentally social in nature, and how individuals relate to others shapes their personality. Many theories (such as those of Heinz Kohut, 2009, and Karen Horney) focus on early social interactions with parents and carers, which are thought to give a grounding that is developed and applied to wider social situations in later life.

However, Erik Erikson (1902–94) considered that personality development continued throughout life into adulthood. He created a 'staged' model of development, with each stage representing a crisis that had to be resolved before the individual could move on to the next stage. Largely speaking, Erikson's theory focuses on the individual finding the solutions to these crises by interacting with others, rather than being the passive recipient of attention.

As it is widely accepted that behaviour is intrinsically linked with surroundings and each individual's social circle, it is self-evident that changing the social structure of the environment will affect behaviour in some way. When considering the behaviour of patients, therefore, not only must we make allowances in terms of what might be considered 'normal' for them in their own sociocultural setting but we must also recognize that, for the duration of the therapeutic relationship, the society in which they find themselves (the hospital) is alien and, therefore, outside their usual normative rules that they are used to and find comfortable.

Stop and think

What aspects of societal behaviour are considered normal in a hospital setting that would not be acceptable in other areas of life? (If you are finding this difficult, you may like to think about the routine questions we ask patients – 'Do you have any false teeth?' or 'When did you last have a bowel movement?')

What impact does environment have on patients' ability to cope?

Erving Goffman (1922–82) did a considerable amount of work on the effects institutions (1968) have on personality (or 'the self' as he described it). His work identified similarities between the populations of prisons and mental hospitals, and he suggested that the culture of institutions has a specific effect on the people who live in them. His view was that institutions change people, and he also warned that the conditions which make prisons 'prison-like' can be found in many other institutions where the residents have broken no laws.

The impacts of rituals and hierarchical management structures on individuals' behaviour can, to a greater or lesser extent, be applied to patients undergoing hospital treatment, and specifically to most patients in operating theatres. In Goffman's terms, the features of an institution include: the processing or treatment of individuals; a clear distinction between inmates (patients) and staff; and the segregation of those under the care of the institution from wider society. All of these criteria are applicable to the perioperative environment at some level and, therefore, that there is some dehumanizing or depersonalization of those subjected to this false society is not difficult to identify.

The effect that Goffman described is discussed extensively by David Lee and Howard Newby (1983), who describe the term 'disculturation' as a progressive process by which the minutiae of the person's pre-admission self are gradually eroded, leaving a personality that will be submissive to the requirements of the institution.

It may not be comfortable to view the standard preoperative processes (such as removing outdoor clothes, wearing a standard hospital gown, being shaved, removing dentures, glasses or hearing aids) in this way – after all, they are in place for a reason – but the effects on the patient's self will be the same, however logical that reason is. Add to this the violation of personal space – in the form of a medical examination or even simply by the application of ECG electrodes or a blood pressure cuff – and being assigned a number, which is checked against a list, over and over again, and it soon becomes evident how effectively such routines can reduce someone with even the most well-balanced personality to feeling like a non-person.

ODPs, unwittingly, can reinforce the norms of institutionalized behaviour when confronted with a busy surgical list and the demands of a theatre team that is under pressure. Unless members of staff are vigilant, the relentless conveyor-belt nature of some theatre lists can surreptitiously influence patient communication to the point where responses become mechanical. Sarafino (2008) describes this phenomenon as staff acting rather like the patient had dropped their body off to them at the repair shop, planning to return to pick it up later. This is a phenomenon in which some patients may appear complicit because they withdraw from the reality of the situation.

The balance of power and control

The changes in what is accepted societal behaviour in a hospital setting mean that healthcare practitioners have an implicit power over the people in their care, something that should not be underestimated. Blaber (2012) counsels that practitioners must be mindful of the potential there is to abuse this power. Society is based on unwritten rules of behaviour that require congruence of roles and responsibilities. Goffman (1990) addressed this concept of society using the analogy of a performance, with the cast taking on specific roles and co-operating together in a performance team.

How do professional roles 'play out' in the operating department?

Goffman suggests that a profession's image with the public may depend on props or costumes, which mark people who have them out as having particular roles – consider how theatre scrubs, masks, stethoscopes and so on identify a member of the operating theatre team. At the same time, specific behaviour is expected of people who are wearing the costumes and using the props. The way in which members of a theatre team behave when setting up for a morning surgical list, with light-hearted banter and conversation, undergoes a seamless transition into professional mode when the patient enters. From this point on, the anaesthetist becomes 'Dr Jones' (before, everyone called him 'Dave'), which expresses to the patient that there is professional respect for members of the team. As Goffman (1990: 166) would assert, 'Backstage familiarity is suppressed'.

Effectively, this places the patient in the position of the audience for the team's performance. However, other sources describe the ease with which patients fall into the role expected of them in a hospital setting. Sarafino (2008) suggests that the environment encourages patients to believe that their involvement in their care is irrelevant – people *learn* to be helpless in hospital. He discusses the concept of staff viewing compliant or passive patients as 'good', while unco-operative or challenging patients are regarded as a problem. A patient who is severely ill may be forgiven for being difficult, but patients who complain when not necessarily suffering significantly may be regarded as troublemakers. Those patients labelled as difficult, in turn, may perceive that they are treated with less compassion than they deserve. Whether or not this really happens does not necessarily change the perception. Patients do not want to antagonize busy members of staff or be thought of as a nuisance, so accept a submissive role to co-operate with them.

Inadvertently, the performance of the professional team underpins the hierarchical difference between the (important) staff and the (lowly) patient (from a patient's perspective), especially if what follows reinforces the imbalance of power in the relationship. By necessity, patients are the passive recipients of actions taken by the members of staff – that is, being a patient requires procedures being 'done to' you. This is counter-intuitive in terms of the basic human instinct of self-preservation, so needs to be handled sensitively.

Patients have expectations of how members of staff will behave in a therapeutic encounter. Practitioners need to comply with the positive aspects of those expectations (of being professional, compassionate, knowledgeable) without reinforcing behaviour that carries a negative connotation (being overbearing, patronizing, overly familiar, inappropriately jovial) in an attempt to make the patient feel as comfortable as possible. Learners in the perioperative environment need to identify which members of the team demonstrate the positive attributes most effectively and work towards emulating effective patient communication. Defining such behaviour or explaining why one member of staff seems to say and do exactly the same as another with very different results requires an understanding of the complex nature of human interaction.

Extending Goffman's theatrical analogy, having the right cast and the right script may result in a believable performance but, equally, may result in a catastrophic medley of unconvincing characters and bad acting. To produce a believable performance the members of the cast need to *inhabit* the characters completely – to *be* the professional, not *act* the professional. This will then enhance the congruence of genuine communication, discussed earlier. The way in which an ODP performs their professional role will change, within given parameters, depending on the interaction they experience with an individual patient. Of course, there has to be a baseline of accepted professional behaviour, but the circumstances of the relationship and the needs of the individual cannot help but affect the outcome of the performance. Flexibility is the key here, and learning to interpret the nuances of the patient's communication is paramount. The aim of any interaction with a patient must surely be to achieve a given purpose for that patient, not to generate a feeling of satisfaction or self-importance in the practitioner that is unrelated to how the patient feels.

Stop and think

Can you identify instances when you or a colleague may have behaved in a particular way to impress a senior member of staff without necessarily considering how that behaviour may have looked to the patient?

Despite advances in patients' rights, there is still an accepted belief among patients that they need to co-operate with the professionals who are looking after them. Implicitly, this allows the practitioner to exercise power over the patient, because the patient is aware of the need to comply with requests made in what they believe will be their best interests.

The nature of power in a therapeutic relationship

Power, in and of itself, is a complex entity to comprehend, leading to a general acceptance of it being dependent on principles of domination and exploitation. Traditionally, power is presented as an object that can be held – or lost. However, philosopher Michel Foucault (1926–84) presented a counterargument about how power works that suggests it is relative rather than concrete. It is not a structure, but a strategy, and it cannot be held, it can only be exercised. Foucault's suggestion (Gauntlett 2008) is that power requires context, and a person who is able to exercise power (not *hold* power) in one setting, such as the chief executive officer (CEO) of a successful company, is not necessarily perceived as powerful in another setting. Foucault asserts that power does not exist outside social relationships, but in relationships it is evident at every level.

Upton (2012) discusses power in the framework of relationships, suggesting that it is the extent to which an individual can persuade another person to act in a certain way. Upton explains that there are various persuasive techniques that individuals may exploit to influence another's behaviour and, of these, 'expert power' – when one party has greater knowledge than the other – is evidently applicable to the practitioner–patient relationship.

If Foucault's model of power relies on reciprocal tacit agreement between the two parties, then the balance of power can be altered by changing the level of control held by each. It is unlikely that a patient will actively try to take control, due to the multifaceted psychological and psychosocial principles outlined earlier in this chapter, which lead them to accept the need for compliance and co-operation. Certainly, in an operating theatre setting, too, the 'powerful experts' will be able to exert total control over the patient's existence in the immediate future, and that is accepted. However, ODPs have the capacity to create balance, by releasing control and gifting power back to the patient. This is a challenging concept. Practitioners are not intentionally wielding power over another weaker individual but, simply by performing their role, they may be creating tensions in patients who experience the very real powerlessness of surrendering to the actions taken by them.

Foucault suggests that, where power exists, resistance is inevitable, and such resistance may be evident as 'quiet tensions and suppressed concern, or spontaneous anger' (Gauntlett 2008: 131). These manifestations mirror the coping strategies of denial and displacement identified by Freud when the id and the superego are in opposition.

Practitioners need to consider whether their communication style is profession-centred or person-centred, and where this places the power in the relationship. For example:

> Hello, my name is Sarah and I shall be looking after you today. I just need to check your name band [picks up arm, reads . . .], 5734628, thank you. Now, I have to attach this monitoring device to you, so that we can keep an eye on all your vital signs while we've got you here today . . .

Most practitioners can identify with these words. On the face of it, the words are friendly and meet the requirement to keep the patient informed of what is going on. On closer examination, however, the power is all focused on the professional 'I am going to do all these things to 'you' and 'you' just have to put up with it.

By reframing the conversation, putting the patient at the centre, the power can be handed back to the patient:

> Hello, Mrs Jones – you are our first patient today. I'm Sarah, and my job is to make sure you are comfortable and cared for while you are with us. Although we need to check a few details with you, I want you to know, you can ask us about anything that you are unsure of, and if you feel uncomfortable about anything, you just have to say and we'll do all we can to make things feel better. Do you mind if I attach these ECG electrodes and blood pressure cuff? Which arm is more comfortable for you?

Of course, the material outcome is the same – the patient is checked in, the necessary procedures are carried out, requirements are met and, in effect, the patient is still at the mercy of the practitioner and the procedure. However, the psychological impact on the patient in the second example is far lower than in the first. Restoring the power, even notionally, to the patient and thereby reducing resistance (consciously or unconsciously) should have a positive effect both on the current procedure and on any future encounters that patient has with the perioperative team.

Stop and think

Rehearse one of your recent patient conversations. Consider how the power balance was being influenced by your words and actions. Could you change the way you approach these conversations to empower patients more effectively?

Psychosocial changes across the lifespan

Much of what has been described so far in this chapter has related to the care of 'a patient' and can, as first principles, be applied to the care of patients across the lifespan. Generally, when considering patient care in operating theatres, 'a patient' is taken to be an adult, although, as this word covers any person over the age of 18, there are going to be considerable differences in the cognitive, experiential and intellectual abilities of all the patients in this category. Also, placing these patients in an unfamiliar environment, under stressful and emotional conditions, is very likely to result in behaviour that may not be considered 'age appropriate'. For this reason, it is not helpful to categorize patients as possessing specific psychosocial attributes by relating their age to the various stages of the human lifespan, as this leads to group definitions that are both unhelpful and (at their core) discriminatory (see under 'Stigma and the group mentality' later in this chapter).

Both cognitive and psychosocial development are continual processes that occur across the whole lifespan, and responses will depend on the internal experiential resources available to any one patient at the time of their surgery rather than their age. Of course, there are some developmental differences that occur at different stages in life, such as those described perhaps most famously by Erik Erikson, but it must be accepted that the boundaries between these stages are not distinct or set, and not every patient will exhibit these kinds of behaviour at any particular stage of their life.

Erikson's theory is based on Freud's psychoanalytical approach, although he does not completely agree with Freud's model. In Erikson's opinion, individual and societal development is a cyclical process, continually affecting and being affected one by the other. Every personal and social 'crisis' provides an experience that will contribute to an individual's emotional or psychological growth. These crises that Erikson describes relate to polar opposite forces that simultaneously challenge humans, on the one hand, to strive, grow and reach out for new experiences and, on the other hand, to retreat to a place of lesser complexity and, by definition, greater comfort (Maier 1978). In Erikson's view, these crises need to be resolved for human beings to achieve fulfilment and, broadly speaking, people's behaviour at different points in the lifespan are associated with different conflicts.

Erikson considers that people are not static products of their upbringing but, rather, are always 'under construction', capable of continually developing and redeveloping, and he describes eight stages of personality development. For example, the earliest conflict is trust versus mistrust, which relates to babies in their first year. For the newborn, a sense of trust requires a feeling of physical comfort, with a minimum amount of uncertainty. Mistrust will arise from unsatisfactory physical experiences (hunger, abandonment) and frustration that may lead to apprehension in later years. The next stage, between one and three years of age, is concerned with developing autonomy versus doubt and shame. Children of this age start to want to make their own decisions and take control of their life. They struggle with the need to develop autonomy, but recognize that this behaviour may alienate them from their carers and, ultimately, leave them defenceless.

General principles for dealing with young people

Caring for paediatric patients in the perioperative environment requires ODPs to have acquired the fundamental understanding that children are not simply small adults. Children do not process information logically or rationally in the same way that adults can, even in familiar and relaxed environments. Hospitalization, and the journey to the operating theatre, presents children with situations that in their home life would be seen as dangerous, frightening and disruptive. They are expected to talk to strangers, agree to situations that appear uncomfortable and out of their control. Even though most paediatric patients are accompanied to theatre by their parents or a primary carer, the emotional toll on those adults creates tensions that the children fail to understand – 'Why is Mummy crying?' 'Why is Daddy scared?' It is worth considering that the prevalence of preoperative parental anxiety can be as high as 74 per cent (Ayenew et al. 2020) and this can increase the likelihood of it being a traumatic experience for the child too (Delgove et al. 2018).

The key to caring for paediatric patients is to ensure the co-operation of the whole perioperative team, and recognize that the surgical list may not be completed on time. This is because the approach required to receive, check in and anaesthetize children for surgery successfully depends on proceeding at a pace that *the child* finds comfortable. Forcing a child to undergo clinical interventions such as cannulation or gaseous induction because the needs of the list are pressing is unacceptable. Being made to co-operate by adults in a position of power can cause significant psychological trauma, which in itself can remain long after the original experience has been forgotten (Martin 2021).

From a power perspective, allowing children the opportunity to make their own choices (within carefully thought out parameters) allows for their autonomy to be acknowledged. Providing the parameters are identified in a suitable way in advance, it makes little difference to the perioperative team whether the child chooses option A or option B, but the psychological advantage of giving control of the situation to the patient will pay dividends. Once the child has invested in the situation by contributing to the decision-making, it is more likely that they will want to be actively involved in the process and be co-operative.

Gaining a child's trust is paramount, and this requires careful handling of the interactions between the clinical members of staff, the primary carer and the patient. Different approaches are required that ostensibly have nothing whatsoever to do with the task in hand. Therapeutic play can be an effective means of reducing preoperative anxiety in children but the evidence to support its efficacy remains inconclusive (He et al. 2015; Silva et al. 2017). Being able to discuss the relative merits of children's television programmes or identify the characters that may be accompanying the child to theatre is a good tactic, but only if it is tackled with sincerity. One thing children are adept at is identifying subterfuge, distraction techniques and insincerity – they have had plenty of experience of being manipulated by parents keen to encourage specific behaviour by bribery or clever questioning!

Things to consider for older adults

At the other end of the lifespan, elderly patients often suffer the indignity of being treated like children, no matter what level of respect they may have commanded throughout their adult life. Age is often described as being nothing more than a state of mind, but Kastenbaum (1979) distinguishes between chronological age, biological age, subjective and functional age, which account for the differences in psychological outlook associated with increasing years. As a person ages, their health requirements (biological age) may dictate an increasing dependence on others to care for their physical needs. The loss of independence – or, in psychological terms, the loss of 'self' – can affect people in several ways, including feeling a loss of identity and decreasing self-worth.

Patients who can recognize their increasing reliance on others fear becoming a nuisance or a burden, which effectively compounds their feeling a loss of engagement with, and usefulness to, society. This may result in them gradually removing themselves from social situations as a source of emotional fulfilment. The fact that this time of life often coincides with people increasingly needing hospital treatment can exacerbate the psychological difficulties that they are experiencing.

Caring for elderly patients, especially in the perioperative environment, may require strategies to deal with their deteriorating physical capabilities. Poor vision, poor hearing and lack of mobility will be evident in many patients. Reduced cognitive abilities may also need to be accommodated, and the incidence of dementia (which is associated with, but not restricted to, patients in the older adult age bracket) is growing across the world. Often patients suffering with dementia become angry and frustrated at their inability to make sense of everyday situations and do everyday things, so stressful encounters with healthcare practitioners are likely to produce extreme behaviour. While compassion, patience and a positive approach may be considered important for all patients, these attributes are paramount when dealing with patients who have lost their in-built psychosocial compass due to the dehumanizing effects of dementia. Despite the salience of compassion for patients with dementia, it is often suboptimal, and this can have a negative effect on patient care and clinical outcomes (Bickford et al. 2019).

Stigma and the group mentality

Earlier in this chapter, Goffman's theories about team performance provided an analogy that helped to explain patient and staff roles. Goffman (1990) also indicated that, backstage, performers often refer to members of the audience using terms that would not be used in face-to-face communication. He suggests a code title may be used that categorizes the audience member (patient) in some way. It is not unusual, for example, to hear a patient being descried as 'the hernia', 'the emergency' or 'the drug user' without this necessarily representing a lack of respect for the individual. It is a practice that arises out of custom or habit rather than intended malice, but doing this fails to take into account what makes each of the patients labelled in this way different from one another. It is dehumanizing, in the sense that the patient is described as an object – a surgical procedure – denying them of their humanness (Rodger and Hartley 2022). This practice is common and perhaps understandable in certain contexts as an adaptive mechanism to protect practitioners by putting psychological distance between themselves and the emotional stress that surgery can cause (Kompanje et al. 2015).

The word 'stigma' is used to describe negative beliefs about something, giving it a devalued social identity (Pescosolido and Martin 2015). People perceived as possessing attributes that have a stigma attached to them may be treated differently from those who do not possess such attributes (Marks et al. 2005). Stigma may be associated with deformity, a disease, an undesirable social history or class, race, ethnicity, religion or belief. The word itself comes from ancient Greek and means a mark or brand.

There have been advances made in legislation that prevents discrimination, with nine protected characteristics being described in the Equality Act 2010, as well as professional ethical guidance that stipulates the need to treat everyone with equal dignity and respect. Despite this, there is a large body of evidence that suggests some practitioners do consciously or unconsciously discriminate, and that this can partially explain health inequalities (Arcaya et al. 2015; Adebowale and Rao 2020).

The habitual labelling of patients with coded titles may also lead to a more widespread 'group mentality', with the practitioner anticipating patients' care needs according to some aspect of their persona that sets them apart in some way. For example, this could be associated with the stigma attached to 'additional needs', 'high risk' or 'elderly'. However, this is inappropriate and demonstrates an inability to recognize the differences that make each person unique.

Stop and think

What assumptions do you make about patients when setting up for an operating list? Do you try to avoid certain theatre sessions that you perceive will present particularly difficult patients? Do you see this as discrimination?

Conclusion

The focus on psychological and psychosocial theories in this chapter should have helped to both highlight and explain the complexities of human behaviour, in general terms and with specific reference to perioperative care. The aim has been to provide ODPs with a foundation for appreciating the breadth of experiences that individual patients bring to the perioperative environment. This chapter has discussed the kinds of common behaviour that may be exhibited by people coming to operating theatres, and highlighted similarities in human experience that occur under specific circumstances. An understanding of these similarities requires a simultaneous acknowledgement of the differences that exist between people. Individuals each bring their own specific baggage to any situation, and while this may be similar to that of others in the same context, this must not be assumed. Clearly, it is not possible to know everything about a patient prior to their hospital visit, and common procedures will follow prescribed patterns for all patients. A skillful ODP will be able to adapt, through effective communication skills and a recognition of the conflicts facing each patient, and so deliver effective, compassionate care that meets the needs of the individual.

Key points

- Patients are affected by their psychological drivers.
- The application of key psychosocial theories to the perioperative environment can be instructive and lead to good practice.
- The hospital experience change the way people behave, which can result in psychological conflict.
- ODPs should be aware of the power balance that exists and understand why this should be handed back to the patient whenever possible.
- Patients should be treated as individuals and not members of groups.

References and further reading

Adebowale, V. and Rao, M. (2020) It's time to act on racism in the NHS, *British Medical Journal*, 368: m568.

Arakelian, E., Swenne, C.L., Lindberg, S., et al. (2017) The meaning of person-centred care in the perioperative nursing context from the patient's perspective: An integrative review, *Journal of Clinical Nursing*, 26: 2527–44.

Arcaya, M.C., Arcaya, A.L. and Subramanian, S.V. (2015) Inequalities in health: Definitions, concepts, and theories, *Global Health Action*, 8(1): Article 27106.

Ayenew, N.T., Endalew, N.S., Agegnehu A.F., et al. (2020) Prevalence and factors associated with preoperative parental anxiety among parents of children undergoing anesthesia and surgery: A cross-sectional study, *International Journal of Surgery Open*, 24: 18–26.

Bandura, A. (1977) *Social Learning Theory*. Upper Saddle River, NJ: Prentice Hall.

Bickford, B., Daley, S., Sleater, G., et al. (2019) Understanding compassion for people with dementia in medical and nursing students, *BMC Medical Education*, 19: Article 35.

Blaber, A. (2012) Psychosocial aspects of health and illness an introduction, in A. Blader (ed.), *Foundations for Paramedic Practice: A Theoretical Perspective*. Maidenhead: Open University Press McGraw-Hill Education.

Bruce, M. and Borg, B. (2002) *Psychosocial Frames of Reference: Core for Occupation-Based Practice*, 3rd edn. Thorofare, NJ: Slack Publications.

Cambridge Dictionary online (2022) Entry for 'care'. Available at: https://dictionary.cambridge.org/dictionary/english/care (accessed October 2022).

Chen, C.S., Chan, S.W., Chan, M.F., et al. (2017) Nurses' perceptions of psychosocial care and barriers to its provision: A qualitative study, *Journal of Nursing Research*, 25(6): 411–18.

Delgove, A., Harper, L., Savidan, P., et al. (2018) How can we decrease preoperative anxiety in parents of children undergoing surgery?, *Archives of Disease in Childhood*, 103(10): 1001–2.

Department of Health and Social Care (DH) (2012) The NHS constitution for England. London: DH. Available at: www.dh.gov.uk/en/Publicationsandstatistics/Publications/PublicationsPolicyAndGuidance/DH_132961 (accessed October 2022).

Etherington, C., Wu, M., Cheng-Boivin, O., et al. (2019) Interprofessional communication in the operating room: A narrative review to advance research and practice, *Canadian Journal of Anesthesia*, 66: 1251–60.

Gauntlett, D. (2008) *Media, Gender and Identity: An Introduction*, 2nd edn. Abingdon: Routledge.

Goffman, E. (1968) *Asylums: Essays on the Social Situations of Mental Patients and Other Inmates*. Harmondsworth: Penguin.

Goffman, E. (1990) *The Presentation of Self in Everyday Life*. Harmondsworth: Penguin.

He, H.G., Zhu, L., Chan, S.W.C., et al. (2015) The effectiveness of therapeutic play intervention in reducing perioperative anxiety, negative behaviors and postoperative pain in children undergoing elective surgery: A systematic review, *Pain Management Nursing*, 16(3): 425–39.

Kastenbaum, R. (1979) *Growing Old: Years of Fulfilment*. London: Harper & Row.

Kohut, H. (2009) *The Restoration of the Self*. London: University of Chicago Press.

Kompanje, E.J.O., Mol, M.M. van and Nijkamp, M.D. (2015) 'I just have admitted an interesting sepsis': Do we dehumanize our patients?, *Intensive Care Medicine*, 41: 2193–4.

Lee, D. and Newby, H. (1983) *The Problem with Sociology*. London: Hutchinson.

Maier, H. (1978) *Three Theories of Child Development*. New York: Harper & Row.

Marks, D. F., Murray, M., Evans, B., et al. (2005) *Health Psychology: Theory, Research and Practice*, 2nd edn. London: Sage.

Martin, R. (2021) *The Management of Procedure-Induced Anxiety in Children*. Cambridge: Cambridge University Press.

Maslow, A. (1970) *Motivation and Personality*, 2nd edn. New York: Harper & Row.

Ockenden, D. (2020) Ockenden report: Emerging findings and recommendations from the independent review of maternity services at the Shrewsbury and Telford Hospital NHS Trust: Our first report following 250 clinical reviews. HC 1081. London: Her Majesty's Stationery Office. Available at: https://assets.publishing.service.gov.uk/government/uploads/system/uploads/attachment_data/file/943011/Independent_review_of_maternity_services_at_Shrewsbury_and_Telford_Hospital_NHS_Trust.pdf (accessed October 2022).

Ockenden, D. (2022) Ockenden report – final: Findings, conclusions and essential actions from the Independent Review of Maternity Services as the Shrewsbury and Telford Hospital NHS Trust. HC 1210. London. Her Majesty's Stationery Office. Available at: www.ockendenmaternityreview.org.uk/wp content/uploads/2022/03/FINAL_INDEPENDENT_MATERNITY_REVIEW_OF_MATERNITY_SERVICES_REPORT.pdf (accessed October 2022).

Pescosolido, B.A. and Martin, J.K. (2015) The stigma complex, *Annual Review of Sociology*, 41: 87–116.

Rodger, D. and Hartley, H. (2022) Understanding intraoperative death, in D. Rodger, K. Henshaw, P. Rawling et al. (eds), *Fundamentals of Operating Department Practice*, 2nd edn. Cambridge: Cambridge University Press.

Rodger, D. and Mahoney, C. (2017) From healthcare assistant to student Operating Department Practitioner: Are you ready for the ODP challenge?, *British Journal of Healthcare Assistants*, 11(5): 248–51.

Rogers, C. (1951) *Client-Centered Therapy: Its Current Practice, Implications and Theory*. London: Constable.

Sarafino, E. (2008) *Health Psychology: Biopsychosocial Interractions*, 6th edn. Hoboken, NJ: John Wiley & Sons, Inc.

Silva, R.D.M. da, Austregésilo, S.C., Ithamar, L., et al. (2017) Therapeutic play to prepare children for invasive procedures: A systematic review, *Jornal de Pediatria*, 93(1): 6–16.

Upton, D. (2012) *Introducing Psychology for Nurses and Healthcare Professionals*, 2nd edn. Harlow: Pearson.

World Health Organization (WHO) (1946) Preamble to the constitution of the World Health Organization. Constitution presented at the International Health Conference, New York, 22 July.

Legislation

Equality Act 2010. Available at: www.legislation.gov.uk/ukpga/2010/15/contents (accessed October 2022).

8 Legal frameworks for Operating Department Practitioners

Helen Booth and Laura Garbett

Key topics

- Understanding the differences between civil and criminal law
- How legal statutes relate to professional practice
- Drug legislation and patient group directions (PGDs)

- Consent
- Confidentiality
- Whistle-blowing
- Conscientious objection to participating in treatment

Introduction

The aim of this chapter is to give Operating Department Practitioners (ODPs) a broad understanding of the legal issues that affect their practice. It is not possible for coverage of the topics to be exhaustive and so, due to the complexities of many of the relevant pieces of law, it is recommended that you also read the references mentioned to gain a more in-depth understanding of this subject.

The law applies to all individuals, though professionals are named where certain requirements apply to them in particular. One good example of this is the Misuse of Drugs and Misuse of Drugs (Safe Custody) Regulations Amendment 2007, in which ODPs are specifically mentioned to give clarity regarding the safe handling of controlled drugs.

This chapter explores legislation pertinent to ODPs and discusses the impacts it has for their role. Examples and discussion points are used as appropriate, but these cannot cover all aspects, so you should relate the content to your own experiences wherever possible.

English law is divided into two distinctive systems – civil and criminal law. All law is derived from the judgments of the courts (common law) or from the legislative work of Parliament. Legislation in the UK generally covers England and Wales, Northern Ireland and Scotland, but it can vary. Therefore, ODPs need to be aware of any variations in the legislation that apply where they are working.

Why is this relevant?

ODPs work in a high-risk area where patients are at their most vulnerable. A sound understanding of professional responsibility, accountability and the legal parameters of their role is therefore essential. The law described in this chapter varies in terms of the impacts it has on individual practitioners. More advanced roles bring with them the need to have a greater depth and scope of understanding of specific legislation and, again, practitioners need to be aware of this. It is paramount that all ODPs keep up to date about changes to legislation (by looking at government websites, for example) as part of their continuing professional development (CPD) and reflect on what impact these may have on their practice. There is no excuse for ignorance of the legal requirements related to the ODP role.

Understanding the differences between civil and criminal law

'Civil law' governs the relationship between individuals and state organizations, covering a vast array of areas. In the context of health, the focus is on the civil law of tort. 'Tort' is the area of law concerned with 'remedies by one person against another in respect of injuries of loss wrongfully caused' (Williams 2006). If one person is found to be liable (the 'defendant'), then the outcome could be, for example, that the defendant needs to pay compensation to the injured party (the 'plaintiff'). The standard of proof in the law of tort is based on the 'balance of probabilities', as opposed to needing to be 'beyond reasonable doubt', which is the case in criminal law. This means the decision-maker must be satisfied that an act or omission was more likely than not to be the cause of the injury or loss.

An important piece of case law that was instrumental in shaping the law of tort is that of *Donoghue* v. *Stevenson* [1932] AC 562. In the case, the 'legal duty of care' was defined and what is known as the 'neighbour principle' by Lord Atkin, who stated that 'you must take reasonable care to avoid acts or omissions which you can reasonably foresee would be likely to injure your neighbour'. Establishing the tort of negligence requires proof that there has been a 'breach of the duty of care' to the claimant. The later case of *Bolam* v. *Friern Hospital Management Committee* [1957] 1 WLR 583 established the 'Bolam test'.

'Criminal law' relates to offences and breaches of statutory law that have negative effects on society as a whole. For the purpose of this chapter, the focus is on those laws that are most applicable to ODPs.

'Statutory law' is made up of all the Acts of Parliament (or statutes), brought into force after a series of procedural steps, create new laws or changes to laws. Statutory law is subdivided into 'primary legislation' and 'secondary legislation. Primary legislation is that which has been passed by Parliament, while secondary legislation is regulations made by means of statutory instruments (Orders, Regulations, Rules, Codes, for example). These laws can see the Crown (referred to as 'R' for 'Regina' or 'Rex' in case law), on behalf of the state, bring a case against a defendant.

The standard of proof required in criminal law is beyond 'reasonable doubt' and, as such, for a guilty verdict, there should be no doubt that the defendant is guilty. If the person is found guilty, this can mean that they need to serve a prison sentence, do community service or another punishment is put in place. In Scotland, there is a further possible outcome, which is 'not proven'.

'Common law' is case law – that is, generally derived from judicial decisions. English law in this area is based on precedent, with courts being obliged to follow previous decisions with relatively well-defined limits. That is why the use of particular cases has driven professional standards and guidelines. Many of these will be discussed in this chapter.

Stop and think

Before proceeding, list the laws that you think have an impact on your individual practice and find out whether these fall into the categories of common, criminal or civil law.

Legal statutes relating to practice

The statutes and related topics discussed in this section include:

- discrimination and the Equality Act 2010;
- consent and the Mental Capacity Act 2005;
- care and the Children's Act 1989 and 2004;
- confidentiality, General Data Protection Regulation 2016 and the Data Protection Act 2018;
- whistle-blowing and the Public Interest Disclosure Act 1998;
- conscientious objection to participating in treatment and the Abortion Act 1967 (Scotland, England and Wales) and Human Fertilisation and Embryology Act (2008);
- samples, organs and tissue donation and the Human Tissue Act 2004 (2006 in Scotland);
- significance to ODPs of the Human Rights Act 1998;
- handling of drugs and the Medicines Act 1968, Human Medicines Regulations 2012 (SI 2012/1916) and the Misuse of Drugs Act 1971.

To ensure clarity, there is a brief description of each Act, followed by its significance to ODPs. Also discussed are points of law on negligence and the Bolam test.

Discrimination and the Equality Act 2010

This Act protects people legally from discrimination in the workplace and in wider society. The previous several anti-discrimination laws – such as the Sex Discrimination Act 1975, Race Relations Act 1976 and Disability Discrimination Act 1995 – were replaced by this single Act, making the law on this subject easier to understand and strengthening protection in some situations (see the Government Equalities Office and Equality and Human Rights Commission guidance, 2013, for more details).

The Equality Act 2010 prohibits discrimination against people with 'protected characteristics', which are specified in section 4 and include:

- age
- disability
- gender reassignment
- marriage and civil partnership
- pregnancy and maternity
- race
- religion
- belief
- sex
- sexual orientation.

Protection from discrimination is afforded to everyone in a variety of situations, including at work, in education, as a consumer, when using public services, buying or renting property or as a member or guest of a private club or association. The Act also protects you if people in your life (such as family and friends) have protected characteristics and you are treated unfairly because of that. This is known as 'discrimination by association'.

ODPs need to be aware that, in the NHS, they are treating patients who are using a public service and, therefore, they should all be treated equally. In the independent sector, although not a public service, the patients are consumers of a service, so have the same rights as patients of the NHS. As an employee, you are afforded the same rights not to be discriminated against under any of the protected characteristics.

As individuals we all have prejudices, whether conscious or unconscious. These could be termed 'personal baggage' and, indeed, we can visualize this like a rucksack on our back. That rucksack, together with the prejudices, needs to be removed while you are carrying out your professional role. Your personal baggage will still be there but, by consciously and physically separating it from you, it should not interfere with how you conduct yourself in your professional practice.

It is the role of all health professionals to challenge other professionals if they become aware of discriminatory or prejudicial behaviour. In most healthcare environments there will be local guidance on how to do this and where and to whom you should take your concerns. Some institutions have created a specific role – known as a 'Freedom to speak up guardian', which is a very important and unique role and offers employees somebody they can speak to if they have concerns. In principle, effectively, failure to challenge discriminatory behaviour is condoning the behaviour. By fostering a culture supportive of challenging such behaviour or prejudices, escalation of workplace bullying can be avoided.

Consent and the Mental Capacity Act 2005

'Consent' is giving permission for something to happen, which may have both legal and ethical dimensions. All adults are presumed to have sufficient capacity to decide on their own medical treatment unless there is significant evidence to the contrary. Valid consent must be obtained before starting treatment, physical investigations or providing personal care to a patient. This reflects the right of patients to determine what happens to their own bodies and is a fundamental part of good practice.

While there is no statute setting out the general principles of consent, common or case law has established that touching a patient without valid consent may constitute the civil or criminal offence of assault and battery. An ODP breaching legal or ethical standards for consent would also be answerable to the regulator of the Health and Care Professions Council (HCPC), having breached its 'Standards of conduct, performance and ethics' (HCPC 2016). The authorities employing the ODP could also be deemed liable for their actions through what is known as 'vicarious liability'. As the employer, they have a supervisory role and so are vicariously responsible for the actions of their employees in the course of their work for them and so, in principle, they would also be liable for the ODP's actions. Furthermore, if the ODP (or any other healthcare professionals) failed to obtain proper consent and the patient subsequently suffered harm as a result of treatment, a claim of negligence may be made against the members of staff involved.

ODPs therefore play a significant role in checking to ensure that the correct consent has been sought. If there is any concern, this should be raised with the multidisciplinary team. Doing this is an example of 'patient advocacy' and this, too, is an exceptionally important part of the work ODPs do.

To assist ODPs in this area, the Department of Health's 'Reference guide to consent for examination or treatment' (2nd ed., DH 2009) provides details of the consent required from patients for physical interventions ranging from major surgery and administering or prescribing drugs to assisting them with dressing. It also sets out clear guidance on who should seek consent and on the subject of the withdrawal and withholding of life-sustaining treatment. It covers adults who do not have the capacity to give consent themselves and gaining consent on behalf of and from children. ODPs need to be responsive to individual situations, know about the differing approaches to consent and consider them in the context of the interventions performed as part of their role.

For consent to be valid, it must be voluntary and informed, and the person consenting must have the capacity to make the decision for themselves. It is far more than simply gaining a signature on a form (which, in fact, isn't a legal requirement). True consent is the result of establishing an open dialogue between yourself and the patient bearing in mind the following key terms.

- **Voluntary:** The decision to consent or not to consent to treatment must be made by the person without any due pressure from family, friends or medical members of staff.
- **Informed:** The person must be given all the information about a treatment and what it involves. All the benefits and risks must be explained and nothing withheld, even when any risk is 1 per cent or less (see *Chester* v. *Afshar* [2004] 3 WLR 927). Alternative treatments should also be discussed. This is usually done by a medical practitioner, as it should be conducted by whoever is undertaking the intervention, but is not necessarily the case.

Stop and think

Before proceeding, what do you think you may require consent for as you undertake your role as an ODP, so you will not potentially commit a civil or criminal offence of battery?

The capacity of the person to understand the information given to them is paramount to them being able to make an informed decision and for their consent to be valid. If the person has capacity and refuses treatment, their decision should be respected, whatever stage of the process they are at. This is still true even if their decision would result in their death or the death of their unborn child.

Consent can be given verbally, non-verbally or in writing and should be obtained in advance, allowing the patient sufficient time to ask questions. Ideally, this should be supported with a written information sheet setting out the procedure. Familiarity with the employing authorities' policy regarding consent and the different consent forms used is essential, as the policy will tie in with the indemnity offered to members of staff as part of their employment. It should be noted that while consent forms are not a legal requirement, they serve to provide evidence of consent. However, if voluntary or informed consent is not gained, then the completion of a consent form becomes irrelevant.

Case law regarding consent

An important case to consider in relation to consent to treatment is *Montgomery* v. *Lanarkshire* [2015] UKSC 11. The plaintiff was pregnant and had insulin-dependent diabetes, which put her at risk of having a larger than average baby. This increased the risk of dystocia by 10 per cent, which can result in the baby's shoulders being unable to pass through the birth canal. The doctor informed Mrs Montgomery that her baby was larger than would be expected for the dates, but failed to warn her about the risk of shoulder dystocia.

When the plaintiff was in labour, shoulder dystocia occurred, resulting in the baby being deprived of oxygen, which led to cerebral palsy in the newborn. When the case first came to court, the Bolam test (see under 'Points of law on negligence and the Bolam test' later in this chapter) was applied to the evidence and the case was dismissed. However, on appeal, the judge concluded that the Bolam test was not applicable and cited as legal precedent and the basis of his decision the case of *Chester* v. *Afshar* [2004] 3 WLR 927. In that case, Lord Walker held that the patient was entitled to information and advice about the possible alternative treatments, which would have been a caesarean section in the *Montgomery* v. *Lanarkshire* case.

When unable to give consent

A patient is considered to lack capacity if their mind is impaired or disturbed in some way that renders them unable to make a decision at that time. Some examples of conditions that may impair a person's ability to give informed consent include:

* dementia
* a severe learning disability
* intoxication from taking drugs or alcohol
* some mental health conditions, such as schizophrenia.

An individual with such an impairment is thought to be unable to make a decision if they cannot:

* understand information relating to the decision;

- remember that information;
- use that information to make a decision;
- communicate their decision.

Patients who lack capacity to make decisions for themselves should not be denied necessary treatment simply because they are unable to give valid consent. The Mental Capacity Act 2005 formalizes the assessment of whether a patient is capable mentally of making such a decision or not, while the Mental Health Acts 1983 and 2007 (amending the 1983 Act) describe the very limited circumstances in which a patient can be forced to be hospitalized for assessment and/or treatment against their wishes. The Mental Health Act 2007 also applies where decisions have to be made on behalf of those who lack the capacity to do so. The decision should always be made with what is best for the patient's personal health and well-being uppermost in everyone's thinking.

In situations that give rise to serious doubt or dispute as to what is in the best interests of an 'incapacitated person', healthcare professionals can refer cases to the Court of Protection for a ruling. Situations that should always be referred to the court include:

- sterilization, for the purpose of contraception;
- the donation of regenerative tissue, such as bone marrow;
- withdrawal of nutrition and hydration from a person who is in a persistent vegetative state;
- where there is serious concern about the person's capacity or best interests.

When a person lacks capacity to give consent, it is essential that the ODP caring for them is aware of the provisions and requirements of the legal statutes and this informs how they approach looking after that patient.

Stop and think

Before proceeding, consider what you would do if you went to a ward to collect a patient and they appeared to be confused about where they were and what was happening to them.

The Mental Capacity Act 2005

Determining 'best interest' under the Mental Capacity Act 2005

The Mental Capacity Act 2005 is complex but many sources of guidance have been developed to help. Dr Theresa Joyce (2007) wrote a document on behalf of the British Psychological Society and it provides clear information and support to members of multidisciplinary teams who may be participating in making decisions on behalf of adults who lack the capacity to do so for themselves. Although the guidance is not specifically aimed at those working in a perioperative environment, it is relevant to ODPs regarding gaining an understanding of the legal issues involved and of patients in this situation when they are participating in their care.

In brief, the guidance raises awareness of the different ways in which people can make decisions on behalf of those who lack the capacity to do so and how the Mental Capacity Act 2005 is relevant to these. It aims to help practitioners who work with individuals who lack the capacity to make their own health decisions, and so need to judge for them what is in their best interest, ensure that they weigh up all the relevant factors as they make those decisions for them. For example, a patient coming into an operating theatre who has a long-term condition, such as Alzheimer's disease, will have gone through a process to establish that the surgery to be performed will be in their 'best interest'. The ODP looking after that patient will, however, still need to check that the records clearly state (as the Association of Anaesthetists for Great Britain and Ireland (AAGBI) 2017, p. 5, advises):

> the grounds on which they have reached this decision, the treatment which will be undertaken, and how this treatment will be in the patient's best interests . . . family members (and, where appropriate, other persons close to the patient) must be consulted when considering patients' best interests, but failure to do so should not compromise care in an emergency.

It is therefore important that the ODP is aware of the considerations that contribute to the 'best interest' decision.

The Act also defines what 'lacking capacity' means. Someone who knows that their capacity to give their consent may be affected in the future may wish to make their wishes known in advance of that happening, recording their decisions (otherwise known as an advance decision or 'living will'), which may help clinicians when the time comes to make treatment choices on their behalf. Such advance decision documents are legally binding in England and Wales so long as they:

- comply with the Mental Capacity Act 2005;
- are valid;
- apply to the situation concerned.

Where an advance decision sets out the desire to refuse life-sustaining treatment, this wish must be written, signed and witnessed, and must include a statement that it applies even when the individual's 'life is at risk'. In Scotland and Northern Ireland, this matter is covered by common law rather than legislation. It will be upheld if the intentions are clear and the adult did not lack capacity at the time it was drawn up.

The National Health Service's (NHS 2020a) information on its website about an advance decision (living will) is something that ODPs may find useful. Although not specifically focused on the perioperative area, it provides good insight into approaches to use when making decisions for others. Areas where this could have impacts on ODPs' practice are in the use of:

- intravenous fluids and parenteral nutrition (tube feeding);
- cardiopulmonary resuscitation;
- life-saving treatment (whether existing or yet to be developed) for specific illnesses that mean capacity or ability to give consent may be impaired, such as brain damage, perhaps from stroke, a head injury or dementia;
- specific procedures, such as a blood transfusion for a patient who is a Jehovah's Witness, because they will have to refuse this treatment as it is against their religious beliefs.

There is also an explanation of the kinds of decisions that should be made.

- **Advance decisions** are those to do with refusing certain treatments and are legally binding, providing they meet certain conditions. If these conditions are met, then they should be implemented, even if they do not appear to be in the best interests of the person who at that point then lacks the capacity to decide.
- **Substituted judgement decisions** are included when the views or wishes of the person when they had capacity are known and must be considered.
- **Best interests decisions** involve weighing up a range of factors (including the wishes or preferences of the person concerned and the views of their families and carers) and deciding what is, on balance, the best for the person, both now and in the future.

Case law regarding mental capacity

It can be helpful to look at some case law on the right to refuse treatment. The two cases described next are well known and the first was cited in the second case as precedence (Kennedy and Grubb 2000).

Re C (adult: refusal of treatment) [1994] 1 All ER 819

This case concerns the right of a competent adult to refuse medical treatment and upholds the principle that mental illness does not automatically call a patient's capacity into question.

C had paranoid schizophrenia and was detained in Broadmoor secure hospital. He developed gangrene in his leg but refused to agree to an amputation, which doctors considered necessary to save his life. The court upheld C's decision for the following reasons:

- the fact that a person has a mental illness does not automatically mean they lack the capacity to make a decision about their medical treatment;
- patients who have capacity (that is, can understand, believe, retain and weigh the necessary information) can make their own decisions to refuse treatment, even if those decisions appear irrational to the doctor or may place the patient's health or their life at risk.

Re MB (adult: medical treatment) [1997] 38 BMLR 175 CA

The focus of this case is on the capacity to refuse treatment.

MB needed a caesarean section, but panicked and withdrew consent at the last moment because of her needle phobia. The hospital obtained a judicial declaration that it would be lawful to carry out the procedure, a decision that MB appealed against. However, she subsequently agreed to the induction of anaesthesia and her baby was born by caesarean section.

The Court of Appeal upheld the judges' view that MB had not, at the time, been competent to refuse treatment, taking the view that her fear and panic had impaired her capacity to take in the information she was given about her condition and the proposed treatment. In assessing the case, the judges reaffirmed the test of capacity set out in the Re C judgment. From this, it can be concluded that:

- an individual's capacity to make particular decisions may fluctuate or be temporarily affected by factors such as pain, fear, confusion or the effects of medication.
- assessment of capacity must be timely and decision-specific.

Wye Valley NHS Trust v. B [2015] EWCOP 60

This case places weight on the beliefs and values of patients who lack capacity.

B required an amputation of his leg, but he was strongly opposed to the operation and had maintained this position for a prolonged period of time. Despite the fact that doctors considered that if B did not have the operation it would lead to his death within days, the Court of Protection found an enforced amputation would not be in B's best interests. The court ruled that proper weight needs to be given to the wishes, feelings and beliefs of those lacking capacity.

The above cases demonstrate the rights of patients and the difficulties these pose for medical practitioners when they are trying either to assess the capacity of patients to make an informed decision or they make decisions seemingly not in their best interests.

Care and the Children's Act 1989 and 2004

The Children's Act 1989 covers all aspects of children's services, including education, welfare and health. The most significant aspect of this act for ODPs is the rights of children to determine their care, especially regarding consent and treating children and their families with respect and safeguarding them.

Due to the complexity of the Act and to provide direction, implementation documents were produced under the National Service Framework (NSF). 'Getting the right start: National Service Framework for children: Standard for hospital services' (DH 2003a) set out a ten-year plan, outlining targets in health and social care to improve services for children. The NSF for children's standard for hospital services (DH 2003a) set out some key aspects that relate to and have an impact on the role of the ODP. For example, the NSF states that 'where care is provided for children there must be staff trained in life support' (DH 2003a: 22). Whereas basic life support is usually sufficient in most surgical recovery and day case facilities, there should be at least one person with a Paediatric Advanced Life Support (PALS) qualification. This also includes the availability of drugs and equipment to stabilize a critically ill child.

All staff who work with children need to ensure that they are 'trained, updated, supported and supervised in safeguarding children and promoting their well-being' (DH 2003a: 23). ODPs should therefore be aware of their professional accountability in relation to having the appropriate knowledge and skills when working with children.

Stop and think

Think of the facilities you have in your department in relation to the children. What training have practitioners undertaken? How would you like to improve the services given to children who come to your operating theatre?

The Children's Act 2004 is a development from the 1989 Act and it reinforced that all people and organisations working with children have a responsibility to help safeguard them and promote their welfare. The Act sets out how a child should be looked after in the eyes of the law and it has an ultimate goal to make the UK a safer place for children. One of the main areas of the Act is the wellbeing of children and the need to make any findings of maltreatment known to the relevant authorities.

Case law regarding children and consent

The first important piece of case law to consider here is that of *Gillick* v. *West Norfolk and Wisbech AHA* [1986] AC 112. In this landmark case, a mother named Victoria Gillick took her local health authority – West Norfolk and Wisbech Area Health Authority – to court to challenge the lawfulness of DH guidance that doctors could provide contraceptive advice and treatment to girls under the age of 16 without parental consent or knowledge in some circumstances.

The House of Lords upheld that a doctor could give contraceptive advice and treatment to a young person under the age of 16 if:

- she had sufficient maturity and intelligence to understand the nature and implications of the proposed treatment;
- she could not be persuaded to tell her parents or to allow her doctor to tell them;
- she was very likely to begin or continue having sexual intercourse with or without contraceptive treatment;
- her physical or mental health were likely to suffer unless she received the advice or treatment;
- the advice or treatment was in the young person's best interests.

Although this case was about contraceptive advice, it has been used as the point in law regarding the capability of children under 16 to consent to treatment. Kennedy and Grubb (2000) note the significance of Lord Scarman's comments in his judgment of the Gillick case in the House of Lords (1985) that are often referred to as the test of 'Gillick competence': the child or young person should be able to understand the nature of the advice and have sufficient maturity to comprehend what is involved. The related 'Fraser guidelines' are those set out by Lord Fraser in his judgment of the Gillick case in the House of Lords (1985).

The Gillick competence test and Fraser guidelines are often used and interchangeable as the premise of both is that it is the right of a child who has sufficient understanding to decide on their treatment or procedure. Awareness of a child's rights in any given situation in the perioperative environment is paramount, particularly their right to refuse treatment. This can give rise to anxiety and frustration for those present, especially the child's parents or carers who, naturally, will feel responsible for the child. ODPs in such situations need to ensure that they are supportive to both the child and the parents or carers and use their skills of empathic communication to ensure the right outcome is achieved. The child's right to refuse does depend on them having sufficient competence and understanding, however, and it is the role of ODPs and other health professionals to provide all the necessary information, assess this and, if reassured of the child's competency and full understanding, to listen, support and respect their decision.

Points of law on negligence and the Bolam test

'Negligence' occurs when there is a failure in the duty of care provided and a patient incurs an injury or some form of damage.

A breach in the duty of care was cited in the case of *Bolam* v. *Friern Hospital Management Committee* [1957] 1 WLR 583, 587. John Bolam had electroconvulsive therapy (ECT) as treatment for depression, but he was not given a muscle relaxant or provided with adequate restraint prior to the ECT being administered, which resulted in him sustaining serious injuries and fractures. The judge stated that the level of skill displayed by the doctor in this case could not be judged against that of an ordinary member of the public, but needed to be judged against the usual standard set by other doctors with specialist skills in this field of medicine. At that time, there was a lack of agreement as to what advice should be given to patients and what procedures should be followed for ECT, so the doctor was judged not negligent as he acted in accordance with practices accepted as proper by a responsible body of other medical professionals with expertise in that particular area. This judgment gave rise to the widely used term the 'Bolam test'.

This benchmark would be true for ODPs using some measure and standard of practice. A judgment of negligence would depend on whether what the ODP did was in accordance with what a reasonable body of fellow ODPs skilled in that practice would feel is appropriate and expected.

Confidentiality, General Data Protection Regulation 2016 and the Data Protection Act 2018

Regarding patient confidentiality, ODPs are bound by the General Data Protection Regulation 2016, Data Protection Act 2018, Department of Health's (DH) NHS codes of practice for confidentiality (DH 2003b; DH 2010) and the Health and Care Professions Council's (HCPC) 'Standards of proficiency: Operating Department Practitioners' (HCPC 2023) and 'Standards of conduct, performance and ethics' (HCPC 2016), plus contracts of employment. It is encompassed by both common and statutory law, and is part of protecting human rights, as seen in the European Convention on Human Rights.

Use of data and General Data Protection Regulation 2016

Consideration must be given to the General Data Protection Regulation 2016 (GDPR), which applies to:

* personal data, which includes a wide range of personal identifiers, in the form of both automated personal data and manual filing systems, so it is important to note that even data which has been pseudonymized can fall within the scope of GDPR;
* sensitive personal data, which includes genetic and biometric data that uniquely identifies an individual.

Article 5 of GDPR requires that personal data is:

- processed lawfully, fairly and in a transparent manner;
- collected for a specified, explicit and legitimate purpose;
- adequate, relevant and limited to what is necessary in relation to the purpose for which it is processed;
- accurate and, where necessary, kept up to date with every reasonable step taken to ensure that incorrect personal data is erased or rectified without delay;
- kept in a form that permits the identification of data subjects for no longer than is necessary for the purposes for which the personal data is processed;
- processed in a manner that ensures appropriate security.

There are six available lawful bases for processing personal information:

- consent
- contract
- legal obligation
- vital interests
- public task
- legitimate interests.

An important element in GDPR is consent and the regulation sets a high standard for consent: it must be unambiguous, involve a clear, affirmative 'opt in', not simply be a 'pre-ticked opt-in box'. Individuals must also be informed of their right to withdraw their consent at any time and be provided with clear and easy ways to do so.

Stop and think

How do you think GDPR affects ODPs, especially from an independent research perspective?

Provisions of the Data Protection Act 2018

Confidentiality is governed by the Data Protection Act 2018 (which supersedes the Data Protection Act 1998), and it clearly states that people have a right to expect the information they give is used only in relation to the purpose for which it was given. They also have a right to control access to their own personal health information, which means ODPs cannot discuss matters relating to patients outside the clinical setting, as they could potentially be overheard, nor leave records unattended, as they may be read by others. Looking through patients' notes should also be on a 'need to know' basis, to inform yourself and others as necessary of any conditions relevant to their care. Although patients have a legal right to gain access to their health records, it is inappropriate to do so in the perioperative environment. All verbal requests should be directed in a way that follows the employing authority's procedure for gaining access to health records.

Confidentiality forms an important part of the trust between health professionals and patients. Patients have a right to privacy, and when they confide their personal details to health professionals, they expect that the information will not be disclosed to others unless required to help with their treatment. The DH's 'Confidentiality: NHS code of practice' (2003b), governed by the original Data Protection Act 1998, has since been superseded by the Data Protection Act 2018, in which it is stated that patients' health information and their interests must be protected by means of the following measures:

* procedures to ensure that all staff, contractors and volunteers are fully aware of their responsibilities regarding confidentiality at all times;
* recording patients' information accurately and consistently;
* keeping patients' information private;
* keeping patients' information physically secure;
* disclosing and using information with appropriate care.

ODPs need to be aware that they should not discuss cases in public areas, particularly operating theatre corridors, in the process of moving and transferring between anaesthetic, surgical and post-anaesthetic areas, and in changing rooms and rest areas. These areas are predominately frequented by other healthcare staff and, at times, the general public. Sharing information is acceptable, however, when seeking advice, sharing an experience or knowledge, but a patient's identity should not be disclosed.

ODPs also need to be aware that key details can easily lead to a person's identity becoming evident, and gossiping is never acceptable. Students and practitioners doing further study should be aware of the pitfalls of breaching confidentiality when writing and sharing experiences and, therefore, students should ensure that they are familiar with and follow their university's confidentiality guidelines.

It is every practitioner's responsibility to keep patients' details secure. This means not leaving patients' details visible and files open on a computer screen, always following the correct procedure for signing out. Medical notes and paper files should never be left unattended or in an easily accessible area. Vigilance between members of a team is essential and making others aware of any potential breach is good practice.

Exemptions and the DH's NHS codes of practice for confidentiality

There are exemptions from the need to maintain confidentiality and these are clearly laid out in the criteria given in the DH's document, 'Confidentiality: NHS code of practice: Supplementary guidance: Public interest disclosures' (2010). This document expands on the principles in the original guidance mentioned earlier in this section, 'Confidentiality: NHS code of practice' (2003b). This supplementary guidance is aimed at supporting staff making difficult decisions about whether disclosures of confidential information may be justified or in the public interest.

Examples of where public interest can be a defence (DH 2010: 9) include:

* reporting to the Driver and Vehicle Licensing Centre a patient who rejects medical advice not to drive (although health professionals should inform the patient of their intention to report this);

- breaching the confidentiality of a patient who refuses to inform their sexual partner of a serious sexually transmissible infection;
- releasing relevant confidential information to social services where there is a potential risk of significant harm to a child.

Whistle-blowing and the Public Interest Disclosure Act 1998

The Public Interest Disclosure Act became law in 1999 and required all NHS trusts and health authorities to have a whistle-blowing policy (DH 1999). The intention of this is to give protection to employees who want to disclose information regarding matters relating to their employment. The protection includes them not being dismissed or penalized by their employers as a result of their disclosure. The whistle-blowing provisions now in place make confidentiality clauses in agreements between workers and employers unenforceable.

Employees intending to use the whistle-blowing provisions need to ensure that their disclosure is for one or more of the following reasons:

- a criminal offence has been committed, is being committed or is likely to be committed;
- a person has failed, is failing or is likely to fail to comply with any legal obligation to which they are subject;
- a miscarriage of justice has occurred, is occurring or is likely to occur;
- the health or safety of any individual has been, is being or is likely to be endangered;
- the environment has been, is being or is likely to be damaged, or information which would reveal something falling into any of the categories listed above has been or is likely to be deliberately concealed.

The circumstances in which you may make disclosures vary depending on the recipient. You should make the disclosure in accordance with your employer's whistle-blowing policy. Such a policy should identify the person you should speak to if you have concerns about taking the information to your employer.

ODPs have a responsibility to act to protect the public, so if you witness and/or have concerns about malpractice in your workplace, the Act will protect you as a 'whistle-blowers' from victimization or dismissal, provided you have have behaved responsibly in dealing with your concerns. For a disclosure to be protected by the law you should make it to the right person, in the right way.

Raising and escalating concerns

At times, concerns may arise, but an ODP does not wish to follow the formal whistle-blowing policy. In this situation, the regulator (HCPC) has set out some guiding principles for raising and escalating concerns regarding another professional's fitness to practice. ODPs in such a situation have a duty to act on concerns as set out in Standard 1 given in the 'Standards of conduct, performance and ethics' (HCPC 2016), which requires us to 'promote and protect the interests of service users and carers'.

The matter should, in the first instance, be brought to the attention of your manager, but if this is not appropriate, a senior manager or Freedom to speak up guardian in the organization. It may be possible to address the matter internally, but if, if for any reason, it is not addressed in a timely manner, then you should take this further up the organization or to the relevant professional regulatory body.

Conscientious objection to participating in treatment and the Abortion Act 1967 (Scotland, England and Wales) and Human Fertilisation and Embryology Act 2008

At times, ODPs may wish to raise a conscientious objection to participating in the treatment being given to a patient. In law, there are two areas where the right to do so is accepted:

- Section 4(1) of the Abortion Act 1967 (Scotland, England and Wales) acknowledges the right to refuse to have direct involvement in abortion procedures;
- Section 38(2) of the Human Fertilisation and Embryology Act 2008 acknowledges the right to refuse to participate in technological procedures to achieve conception and pregnancy.

In any legal proceedings, the burden of proof of conscientious objection will be with the person claiming to rely on it.

However, the Abortion Act 1967 does place a caveat in Section 4(2): 'Nothing . . . shall affect any duty to participate in treatment which is necessary to save the life or to prevent grave permanent injury to the physical or mental health of a pregnant woman', even Section 4(1). This means that in the case of an emergency, you have a duty to participate and not omit the care required, to act in the best interests of the patient.

Any ODP who wishes to make it known that they are a conscientious objector regarding one or more particular treatments should speak with a senior member of staff and follow this up in writing, stating that they do not wish to participate in that or those practices. The ODP should do this as soon as possible and certainly well in advance of the possibility of being in such a situation. It would be unacceptable to do so once a patient has presented as it may cause staffing and care delivery issues that could result in harm to the patient.

Stop and think

As an ODP in charge of a surgical list, how would you handle the following situation?

Your team is short-staffed due to sickness. A health professional has been assigned to your surgical list at short notice by a senior member of staff. It is only once they have arrived that they realize the list they have been asked to work on is a very busy termination of pregnancies list. The health professional informs you that they cannot participate in the team for this list as they are a conscientious objector and put this in writing some time ago.

Samples, organ and tissue donation and the Human Tissue Act 2004 (2006 in Scotland)

The removal of products, specimens and samples is common practice in operating theatres and, therefore, the Human Tissue Act 2004 (2006 in Scotland) is relevant to the activities of ODPs. The Act regulates how the removal, storage and use of human tissue from either the living or dead is organized and controlled. This includes any organs or residual tissue following clinical and diagnostic procedures. The Act also makes consent a legal requirement for the removal, storage and use of human tissue or organs and sets out whose consent is needed in which circumstances.

The Human Tissue Authority (HTA) is the licensing body responsible for approving the transplantation of organs from living donors, including bone marrow and peripheral blood stem cells from adults who lack the capacity to give their consent and children who lack the competence to do so themselves. The HTA also licenses activity regarding stem cells and how they are removed, stored and processed. Since 2008, anybody collecting cord blood needs to have a licence to do so from the HTA. This covers the collection, quality of the samples and how they are stored, consent of the mother and lawful use of the samples. ODPs may see this following a caesarean section where it is the wishes of the parents that such samples be collected.

Significance to ODPs of the Human Rights Act 1998

The Human Rights Act 1998 is a law that has as its core values fairness, respect, equality and dignity. It came into force in the UK in October 2000 and includes the rights enshrined in the European Convention on Human Rights. Despite Brexit, the 1998 Act is still applicable to the UK and the government is still obliged to ensure that the rights detailed in the Act are protected. Section 2 of the Act interprets the rights of the European Convention, and Section I, Article 2 of the European Convention itself is most significant to the role of the ODPs as it deals with the right to life, so relates to issues such as do not resuscitate orders, refusal of life-saving medical treatment, advance directives (or living wills) and death through negligence.

Although Article 2 of the Convention is the most significant, the other main articles are also relevant in medical law are:

- **Article 3** prohibiting torture and inhuman or degrading treatment or punishment;
- **Article 5** the right to liberty and security;
- **Article 8** the right to respect for private and family life;
- **Article 9** the right to freedom of thought, conscience and religion;
- **Article 12** the right to marry and found a family;
- **Article 14** the prohibition of discrimination so as to enjoy the rights set out in the Convention rights.

In healthcare, abiding by the Human Rights Act is all about balancing different people's rights and often (DH and BIHR 2008):

> rights appear to conflict with each other, judgements have to be made about priorities or boundaries. There are many instances in NHS organisations where rights have to be balanced to protect the safety or rights of others, or in the

interests of good order. For example, ensuring that staff are protected from violent or abusive patients while also having regard to the interests of the patient.

Stop and think

Before proceeding, consider how the 'recommended summary plan for emergency care and treatment' (ReSPECT; Resuscitation Council UK n.d.) fits with Article 2 of the European Convention on Human Rights – the right to life.

Handling of drugs and the Medicines Act 1968, Human Medicines Regulations 2012 (SI 2012/1916) and the Misuse of Drugs Act 1971

Handling drugs is very much part of the role of an ODP. Therefore, knowledge and understanding of the legislation concerning this subject is paramount as ignorance is no defence in the eyes of the law. Changes occur to the regulations and legislation over time and it is essential that ODPs' knowledge remains current by checking regularly for news of updates and new information.

The Medicines Act 1968

The Medicines Act 1968 is the guiding legislation, controlling the manufacturing and distribution of medicinal products. It is often referred to as primary legislation and cross-references to it when there are amendments or further regulations are developed. The significance of the Act is that it sets out the legal status of drugs and their classifications regarding penalties.

Each medicinal product is given a legal status and this correlates to how the medicines can be supplied.

- on prescription referred to as prescription-only medicines (POMs);
- in a pharmacy without prescription, under the supervision of a pharmacist (P);
- on general sale (GSL), so can be sold in general retail outlets without the supervision of a pharmacist.

Prescriptions can be issued by doctors, dentists, regulated professional independent prescribers, pharmacist independent prescribers and supplementary prescribers.

The regulation of medicines is the responsibility of the Medicines and Healthcare Products Regulatory Agency (MHRA), which is also responsible for medical devices and equipment used in healthcare, plus the investigation of harmful incidents. The MHRA also has responsibility for blood and blood products, working with UK blood services, healthcare providers and other relevant organizations to improve blood quality and safety. It provides excellent online information for practitioners working in operating theatres, such as guidance, safety alerts and interactive educational material.

While the Medicines Act gives the overarching framework for drug legislation, the piece of legislation most familiar to ODPs is the Misuse of Drugs Act 1971 governing controlled drugs.

The Human Medicines Regulations 2012 (SI 2012/1916)

These regulations set out a comprehensive regime for the authorization of products for manufacture, import, distribution, supply and sale. They introduced a small number of policy changes to ensure that the legislation is fit for purpose and include some exceptions for health professionals, which may be relevant to ODPs with an advanced scope of practice. In particular, Part 3.9 specifies that 'Persons who hold the advanced life support provider certificate issued by the Resuscitation Council (UK) may administer Adrenaline 1:10,000 up to 1mg; and amiodarone'. However, this 'shall only be in an emergency involving cardiac arrest'.

The Misuse of Drugs Act 1971

The Misuse of Drugs Act 1971 is divided into regulations that have as part of them the classification related to the misuse of drugs, the scheduling of drugs and the safe custody. The misuse classification of drugs in the UK is set out in three classes – Classes A, B and C – which relate to the risk of harm the drugs pose to individuals or to society by their misuse. Class A drugs pose a very high risk of harm (heroin, cocaine, methadone, ecstasy, lysergic acid diethylamide, known as LSD or acid, and magic mushrooms). Class B drugs less harm (these include amphetamines, barbiturates, codeine, cannabis and synthetic cannabis). Class C drugs less harm still (these include benzodiazepines, which are tranquillizers, gamma-hydroxybutyrate, known as GHB, anabolic steroids, gamma-butyrolactone, known as GBL, and benzylpiperazines).

The classifications and type of misuse of these drugs are reflected in the periods of sentencing and fines incurred. These vary depending on the class of drug and whether it was only in the person's possession or there was also an intent to sell it. The quantity of drugs involved, any previous criminal record and the circumstances of the offence or offences will also influence the outcomes.

The scheduling of drugs is controlled by the Misuse of Drugs Regulations 2001, which divides drugs into five schedules, and these correspond to their potential for being therapeutic, useful or misused. A number of changes affecting the prescribing, record-keeping and destruction of controlled drugs have been introduced as a result of amendments to the Misuse of Drugs Regulations 2001. In 2006, amendments were made in response to safe management of medicines and, in 2007, an amendment was made (resulting in the Misuse of Drugs and Misuse of Drugs (Safe Custody) (Amendment) Regulations 2007) giving authority to ODPs to possess and supply controlled drugs, which previously only senior registered nurses could do (see also Home Office 2007).

The schedules relate to the recording, administration and disposal of a drug. ODPs are accountable for keeping clear, timely and correct records of drugs they supply to medical practitioners or independent prescribers. The drugs mentioned as examples in the following list of the schedules are the ones that ODPs will have most exposure to in operating theatres and related areas:

- **Schedule 1:** drugs that have no recognizable medical use, such as raw opium and hallucinogens;

- **Schedule 2:** pharmaceutical opiates, used during and post anaesthesia, for which a register must be kept (all Schedule 2 controlled drugs need to be entered) and this register must comply with the relevant regulations;
- **Schedule 3:** barbiturates;
- **Schedule 4:** benzodiazepines;
- **Schedule 5:** drugs given in Schedule 2 but at a lesser concentration, such as cocaine paste.

In the event that ODPs have to dispose of a residual amount of a drug, such as may be left in a syringe following an operation, they must do so in accordance with the procedures put in place by their employing authority. There are also the National Institute for Health and Care Excellence (NICE) guidelines, 'Controlled drugs: Safe use and management' (2016), on the destruction of controlled drugs. Any medicines should be disposed of in relevant waste containers that are then sent for incineration and should not be disposed of in the sewerage system. All controlled drugs in Schedules 2, 3 and 4 (part I) can be placed in waste containers only after the controlled drug has been rendered irretrievable (that is, by denaturing). Again, the local policy and best practice need to be followed.

ODPs can administer any prescribed drug in Schedules 2, 3 and 4, or any drug under the directions of a medical practitioner. Many employing authorities have intravenous drug administration training programmes that staff have to undertake if they are to be covered by a local policy. All ODPs should gain access to these to ensure that they comply with the vicarious liability of the employing authority.

As many ODPs are in regular contact with drugs as part of their role, it is paramount that their knowledge remains current and that they keep up to date regarding changes to any of the regulations. It is important to recognize that a medicine or device may hold a product licence, but should there be any change – such as to the strength of a drug or to the use of a piece of equipment – responsibility for the quality of their use will lie with the healthcare professional giving that medicine or using the device, whether that person is an ODP or a medical practitioner.

Potential amendments to the Human Medicines Regulations and Misuse of Drugs Regulations specific to ODPs

The proposed changes to medicines legislation requires amendments to be made to both the Human Medicines Regulations and the Misuse of Drugs Regulations. As a result of the Chief Professions Officers' medicines mechanisms programme of work, NHS England led a consultation on behalf of the four nations of the UK that included changes to responsibilities regarding medicines for ODPs, to enable them to supply and administer medicines under a 'patient group direction' (PGD). The consultation ran from October 2020 to December 2020, but due to the impact of the COVID-19 pandemic, full approval is yet to be received on amendments to legislation that will apply throughout the UK and in any settings where ODPs work and PGDs are permitted (NHS 2020b).

Stop and think

A patient in your care has a high national early warning score (NEWS) and is triggering for 'red flag sepsis'. Consider how a PGD could help with the early management of this situation, in line with NICE guidance.

Key aspects of the legislation are that it specifies each PGD (MHRA 2017) must contain the following information:

- name of the business to which the direction applies;
- date the direction comes into force and the date it expires;
- description of the medicine(s) to which the direction applies;
- class of health professional who may supply or administer the medicine;
- signature of a doctor or dentist, as appropriate, and a pharmacist;
- signature by an appropriate member of the health organization;
- clinical condition or situation to which the direction applies;
- description of the circumstances in which further advice should be sought from a doctor (or dentist, as appropriate) and arrangements for referral;
- details of appropriate dosage and maximum total dosage, quantity, pharmaceutical form and strength, route and frequency of administration, and minimum or maximum period over which the medicine should be administered;
- relevant warnings, including potential adverse reactions;
- details of any necessary follow-up action and the circumstances;
- statement of the records to be kept for audit purposes.

Any changes to the legislation would mean that all registered ODPs would be eligible to supply and administer medicines using PGDs, subject to local governance. ODPs would need to ensure that they were aware of the local policy in relation to the use of PGDs. Access would need to be made available for healthcare staff to local training programmes or the e-learning through NHS England (NHS England and Specialist Pharmacy Service n.d.).

Conclusion

The legislation discussed in this chapter represents the key areas that have impacts on ODPs' working practice. The role of ODPs has changed and developed over the years and with this has come greater responsibility and accountability regarding understanding the areas of the law that relate to their scope of practice. Many of these are translated into the policies and procedures of your employing authority.

The overview of the law given in this chapter serves to direct ODPs to the legal fundamentals related to their role. It is part of that role to keep updated about any changes that affect ways of working and so on. Reading widely about and around your area of practice is both necessary and invaluable, particularly for those in an advanced role.

Key points

- It is essential that ODPs develop their understanding of legal terms and how they affect their practice.
- ODPs are responsible and accountable for consent and confidentiality, and handling these correctly is key to upholding the rights of patients.
- To fulfil their role, ODPS need to have a clear understanding of the drug legislation and it is their responsibility to remain up to date regarding any changes so their knowledge is current.

References and further reading

Association of Anaesthetists for Great Britain and Ireland (AAGBI) (2017) Consent for Anaesthesia. London: AAGBI. Available at: https://anaesthetists.org/Portals/0/PDFs/Guidelines%20 PDFs/Guideline_consent_for_anaesthesia_2017_final.pdf?ver=2018-07-11-163753-600&ver=2018-07-11-163753-600 (accessed November 2022).

Department of Health (DH) (1999) Public Interest Disclosure Act 1998: Whistleblowing in the NHS. Health Services Circular HSC 1999/198. London: DH.

Department of Health (DH) (2003a) Getting the right start: National Service Framework for children: Standard for hospital services. London: DH. Available at: https://assets.publishing.service.gov.uk/government/uploads/system/uploads/attachment_data/file/199953/Getting_the_right_start_-_National_Service_Framework_for_Children_Standard_for_Hospital_Services.pdf (accessed November 2022).

Department of Health (DH) (2003b) Confidentiality: NHS code of practice. London: DH. Available at: www.gov.uk/government/publications/confidentiality-nhs-code-of-practice (accessed October 2022).

Department of Health (DH) (2009) Reference guide to consent for examination or treatment, 2nd edn. London: DH. Available at: www.gov.uk/government/publications/reference-guide-to-consent-for-examination-or-treatment-second-edition (accessed October 2022).

Department of Health (DH) (2010) Confidentiality: NHS code of practice: Supplementary guidance: Public interest disclosures. (Extends the DH's 'Confidentiality: NHS code of practice', 2003b.) London: DH. Available at: www.gov.uk/government/publications/confidentiality-nhs-code-of-practice (accessed October 2022).

Department of Health (DH) and British Institute of Human Rights (BIHR) (2008) Human rights in healthcare: A framework for local action, 2nd edn. London: DH. Available at: www.choiceforum.org/docs/hrframe.pdf (accessed October 2022).

Government Equalities Office and Equality and Human Rights Commission (2013) Equality Act 2010: Guidance. London: Government Equalities Office and Equality and Human Rights Commission. Available at: www.gov.uk/equality-act-2010-guidance (accessed October 2022).

Health and Care Professions Council (HCPC) (2016) Standards of conduct, performance and ethics. London: HCPC.

Health and Care Professions Council (HCPC) (2023) Standards of proficiency: Operating Department Practitioners. London: HCPC.

Home Office (2007) Home Office Circular (027/2007): Misuse of Drugs and Misuse of Drugs (Safe Custody) (Amendment) Regulations 2007. London: Home Office. Available at: www.gov.uk/government/publications/misuse-of-drugs-and-misuse-of-drugs-safe-custody-amendment-regulations-2007 (accessed November 2022).

Joyce, T. (2007) Best interests: Guidance on determining the best interests of adults who lack capacity to make a decision (or decisions) for themselves (England and Wales). Leicester: Professional Practice Board of the British Psychological Society, funded by the Department of Health. Available at: www.scie.org.uk/publications/guides/guide03/files/bestinterestsguide. pdf?res=true (accessed October 2022).

Kennedy, I. and Grubb, A. (2000) *Medical Law*, 3rd edn. Oxford: Butterworth.

Medicines and Healthcare Products Regulatory Agency (MHRA) (2017) Patient group directions: Who can use them. London: MHRA. Available at: www.gov.uk/government/publications/ patient-group-directions-pgds/patient-group-directions-who-can-use-them (accessed October 2022).

National Health Service (NHS) (2020a) Advance decision to refuse treatment (living will): End of life care. London: NHS. Available at: www.nhs.uk/conditions/end-of-life-care/advance-decision-to-refuse-treatment (accessed October 2022).

National Health Service (NHS) (2020b) Consultation on the proposal for the supply and administration of medicines using patient group directions by Operating Department Practitioners across the United Kingdom. London: NHS. Available at: www.england.nhs.uk/wp-content/ uploads/2020/10/odp-full-consultation-.pdf (accessed October 2022).

National Institute for Health and Care Excellence (NICE) (2016) Controlled drugs: Safe use and management. NICE guideline [NG46]. Manchester: NICE. Available at: www.nice.org.uk/guidance/NG46/chapter/Recommendations#handling-controlled-drugs (accessed October 2022).

NHS England and Specialist Pharmacy Service (n.d.) Patient Group Directions e-learning programme. London: NHS England. Available at: www.e-lfh.org.uk/programmes/patient-group-directions (accessed October 2022).

Resuscitation Council UK (n.d.) ReSPECT. Available at: www.resus.org.uk/respect (accessed October 2022).

Williams, G. (2006) *Learning the Law*, 13th edn. Edinburgh: Sweet & Maxwell.

Legislation and cases

Legislation

Abortion Act 1967: www.legislation.gov.uk/ukpga/1967/87/contents (accessed October 2022).

Children's Act 1989: www.legislation.gov.uk/ukpga/1989/41/contents (accessed October 2022).

Children's Act 2004: www.legislation.gov.uk/ukpga/2004/31/contents (accessed October 2022).

Data Protection Act 2018: www.legislation.gov.uk/ukpga/2018/12/contents/enacted (accessed November 2022).

Equality Act 2010: www.legislation.gov.uk/ukpga/2010/15/contents (accessed November 2022).

European Convention on Human Rights: www.echr.coe.int/documents/d/echr/convention_ENG (accessed November 2022).

General Data Protection Regulation 2016 (Regulation (EU) 2016/679 of the European Parliament and of the Council, commonly known as GDPR): www.legislation.gov.uk/eur/2016/679/contents (accessed November 2022).

Human Fertilisation and Embryology Act 2008: www.legislation.gov.uk/ukpga/2008/22/contents (accessed November 2022).

Human Medicines Regulations 2012: www.legislation.gov.uk/uksi/2012/1916/contents/made (accessed November 2022).

Human Rights Act 1998: www.legislation.gov.uk/ukpga/1998/42 (accessed October 2022).

Human Tissue Act (2004) (Scotland 2006): www.legislation.gov.uk/ukpga/2004/30/contents (accessed October 2022).

Medicines Act 1968: www.legislation.gov.uk/ukpga/1968/67 (accessed October 2022).

Mental Capacity Act 2005: www.legislation.gov.uk/ukpga/2005/9/contents (accessed October 2022).

Mental Health Act 1983: www.legislation.gov.uk/ukpga/1983/20/contents (accessed October 2022).

Mental Health Act 2007 (amending the 1983 Act): www.legislation.gov.uk/ukpga/2007/12/contents (accessed October 2022).

Misuse of Drugs Act 1971: www.legislation.gov.uk/ukpga/1971/38/contents (accessed October 2022).

Misuse of Drugs and Misuse of Drugs (Safe Custody) (Amendment) Regulations 2007: www.legislation.gov.uk/uksi/2007/2154/made (accessed October 2022).

Misuse of Drugs Regulations 2001: www.legislation.gov.uk/uksi/2001/3998/contents/made (accessed October 2022).

Public Interest Disclosure Act 1998: www.legislation.gov.uk/ukpga/1998/23/contents (accessed October 2022).

Cases

Bolam v. *Friern Hospital Management Committee* [1957] 1 WLR 583, 587.

Chester v. *Afshar* [2004] 3 WLR 927.

Donoghue v. *Stevenson* [1932] SC (HL).

Gillick v. *West Norfolk and Wisbech Area Health Authority* [1985] AC 112 (HL).

Montgomery v. *Lanarkshire* [2015] UKSC 11.

Re C (adult: refusal of treatment) [1994] 1 All ER 819

Re MB (adult: medical treatment) [1997] 38 BMLR 175 CA

Wye Valley NHS Trust v. *B* [2015] EWCOP 60

Ethics for Operating Department Practitioners

9

Helen Booth and Rebecca Daly

Key topics

- Why the subject of ethics is relevant to Operating Department Practitioners (ODPs)
- The impact of ethical theories on ODPs' practice

- Understanding guiding principles and approaches to standards of behaviour
- How values and advocacy play a part in working practice
- A framework of questions to use to support and resolve ethical issues

---

Introduction

The professionalization of operating department practice, changes in healthcare and the introduction of advanced roles have meant that practitioners face increasingly complex situations and difficult decisions in their practice. There is the very real possibility of moral burnout if they are not prepared adequately by acquiring the skills of ethical decision-making. The ability to manage the emotional burden of working in a pressurized environment is an expectation set out in the Health and Care Professions Council's 'Standards of proficiency for Operating Department Practitioners' (HCPC 2023). In this chapter we explore the ethical theories and approaches that can contribute to shaping, guiding and underpinning the decision-making process that can make all the difference to ODPs in the complex landscape of critical care.

The key areas explored are the leading theories of Western moral philosophy, the principles that guide standards of behaviour, and decision-making in practice. We also consider how ODPs engage with other health professionals, ensuring that a collective approach to the care of patients is established. The professional regulatory standards and guidelines are not discussed in detail here as, although they act as a useful reference point, they are founded on good professional experience and influenced by legal statutes, which are not our focus in this chapter.

Why is this relevant?

Ethics is a branch of philosophy that is devoted to the study of morality, so it is also called moral philosophy (Newham and Hawley 2007). Ethics itself has several branches, including normative ethics, which provides theoretical frameworks that guide standards of behaviour and tell us how human beings ought to act in many situations, especially in professional roles. Another branch, known as applied ethics, moves beyond theoretical constructs and attempts to identify the moral significance of specific situations. As part of their professional role, ODPs will inevitably have to consider the ethical implications of care and the landscape in which it is delivered. An understanding of normative theories is essential for ODPs as this enables them to engage with applied ethics during such times in clinical decision-making.

The terms 'ethics' and 'morality' both refer to what is right or wrong, but there is a distinction between them. The term 'ethics' refers to frameworks, principles or guides, so, for example, healthcare professionals follow a code of ethics and philosophers refer to theories such as utilitarianism. Morals, however, are associated with personal beliefs about what is right or wrong and, although shaped by different factors, such as culture, these beliefs may clash with ethical frameworks. ODPs need to recognize the distinction between ethics and morals so that they can set aside their personal moral convictions when faced with an ethical dilemma and use objective critical reasoning. This distinction also helps when it comes to differentiating between a moral disagreement and a true ethical dilemma.

Consider a practitioner who believes that a patient's refusal of treatment is morally wrong based on their own belief that life is sacred. The practitioner's belief is not sufficient grounds on its own to constitute an ethical dilemma. Rather, it constitutes a moral disagreement. In cases such as this, it is important that ODPs can identify what their own moral convictions are, as then they can assess whether a true ethical dilemma exists. Unless there are wider factors relevant to this situation, or legal grounds for conscientious objection, in such a case the ODP must respect the wishes of their patient. Factors that may turn the example into an ethical dilemma could include difficulties in ascertaining the patient's mental capacity or if there has been coercion and some familial dispute is involved.

Before exploring ethics in further detail, it is useful to clarify what it is not. Ethics is not:

- simply about feelings, although they do often play a part in ethical dilemmas and should be acknowledged as part of the decision-making process, in terms of their origin – such as the moral agent's personal, religious or cultural beliefs;
- specific to a particular culture, religion or tradition – individual ethical theories are constructed based on different perspectives on what is of normative value, determined by the social and historical constructs that were relevant during their development;
- about following the law, although there are references to standards of behaviour;
- a science, as it cannot always be quantified and measured, although ethics in science is important, particularly in the context of research.

Many would consider ethics to be mere 'common sense', but common sense is usually founded on experience and personal beliefs. However, beliefs and norms are not universal, so it is important to make a distinction between what are personal beliefs, which may or may not align with those of others, and common sense, which is accepted as a standard by most reasonable people most of the time.

When entering a profession and meeting ethics in professional life for the first time, you will often hear people say, 'Isn't that obvious?' or 'Isn't that just common sense?' Such responses are understandable, but it is important to remember that those impressions are based on the learnt behaviour acquired in a particular individual's culture, from their social experience and their peers. Obviously this is of value and forms the basis of most ethical frameworks, but as an approach it is not sufficient, nor structured enough, to be able to deal with the wide variety of complexities encountered in healthcare situations generally and the daily complexities of dealing with patients and colleagues in the perioperative environment. In clinical care, there can often be competing views on what is morally right, and it is this type of situation that constitutes a moral dilemma. For this reason, ethics is an integral part of professional life and, therefore, practitioners are required to develop their understanding of this subject area and the value of using ethical frameworks to underpin and guide their critical reasoning.

The different ethical theories provide a framework for debate, discussion, disagreement and understanding. Several of these theories and approaches, all of which are derived from traditional Western moral philosophy, are explained in the next section, so it is clear what the main points of these debates are. Although at first they may not seem relevant to everyday situations, you will find that they do help with difficult decision-making in practice. ODPs now operate in such varied healthcare settings that it is impossible to address all the ethical problems and dilemmas you might be faced with. However, a framework of questions has been developed for this chapter for you to use as an aid to applying critical reasoning to ethical dilemmas in practice.

In healthcare, the various ethical standards are well founded in codes and guidance. They prescribe what practitioners should or should not do, usually in terms of rights, obligations, benefits to the patients and the upholding of specific virtues. The basis for those ethical standards, the thinking of relevant philosophers and how all this relates to ODPs are discussed in the rest of this chapter.

Ethical theories and approaches

The following section examines the classical theories of Western moral philosophy relevant to the practice of ODPs with some examples of how these translate to practical matters. The theories covered here are virtue ethics, deontology and consequentialism. This is followed by consideration of the 'four principles' approach, which has guided professional ethical standards for around 30 years. There are many more ethical approaches but none as well known for their application to practical issues and the values they represent.

In ethical dilemmas, ODPs are faced with choosing an action that will have an effect on someone or something to obtain a specific outcome. Therefore, the theoretical frameworks presented are organized according to this Aristotelian idea of a line of causation. The normative features are the agent (decision-maker), action (the decision) and outcome (impact of the decision). Just as the agent, action and outcome are all necessarily linked, the theories in ethical decision-making each have something to offer in assessing the ethical dimensions of a dilemma.

The normative feature of each theory also becomes its limitation when taken in isolation. For this reason, ethical theories are not to be seen as mutually exclusive when applied to ethical dilemmas and clinical decision-making. Instead, they are used together to offer perspective.

Virtue ethics

Virtue ethics originates from the work of Greek philosopher Aristotle (van Hooft 2006) and centres on the character of the moral agent. Aristotle believed that all objects have a purpose, or *telos*, including human beings. Just as the *telos* of a chair is to function as a 'good' chair, the *telos* of human beings is to do things conducive to happiness, or *eudaemonia*, through acting in a virtuous way in accordance with reason. *Eudaemonia* has been translated as both happiness and flourishing. Achieving the virtues, or excellences of character, requires the moral agent to employ *phronesis*, which translates as practical or moral wisdom. Experience and habituation are necessary to become virtuous.

To be of virtuous character requires us to steer a good middle path rather than veer towards deficiency or excess. For example, a virtuous moral agent may act from courage but never rashness or cowardice. In deciding what it is morally right to do, a moral agent should be guided by what morally right action a virtuous person would take. Employing practical wisdom is what allows a moral agent to identify that which makes their actions virtuous. For this reason, virtue ethics sets itself aside from theories that favour following rules out of duty or those which do not consider the emotional response of the agent.

The agent-centred nature of virtue ethics does, however, also become its limitation, as its focus places the normative value in any situation as the agent acting virtuously. It does not place emphasis on the moral nature of the action itself or the outcome, although they are still integral. Further, there is a disregard for general principles or norms, which means that there is little external guidance regarding what actions a virtuous person would take.

Regarding ODPs and wider multidisciplinary teams (MDTs), virtue ethics can be applied to the practice of upholding the qualities required of a professional practitioner. With changes to views on values in the health service, efforts have been made to bring virtue theory back into focus on this very point, with the aim of framing the characteristics of professionals as ones that have a moral significance in their caring role. Employing their accrued wisdom, alongside experience, allows practitioners to demonstrate virtue in their practice.

Deontology (duty-based ethics)

The best-known advocate and the founder of duty-based ethics was Immanuel Kant (1724–1804). His theory is that if an action is correct, it is correct regardless of the harm or benefits it may produce. Kant ([1785] 1964) believed that it is feasible to develop a consistent moral system by using reason. The idea is that there are particular duties that must be upheld at any cost – unconditional moral laws that can be applied to all rational beings. Kant prescribes the 'categorical imperative' as a way of determining logically, using our reason, what is right and wrong – it tells us what we ought to do. He suggested three ways in which this could be carried out:

- do things in such a way that your actions can and ought to be universal;
- treat people as ends in themselves and never solely as the means to an end;
- act as you would have someone act towards you.

According to duty ethics, therefore, you could not justify an action purely on the basis that it produces a good outcome. The emphasis is on valuing each human being and showing equal respect to all.

Kant's theory of the categorical imperative became the foundation for his 'principles' approach to ethics, which lies in the 'respect for persons'. It is arguable that this principle can apply to all aspects of life, whether it be health or other factors, but it is only right that each individual is worthy of respect, whether we like them or not. It provides the foundation for how we should treat others. Indeed, potentially it could be the only overarching principle and value needed for all professionals in a given work situation and it sits well with the value all should afford to both our patients and colleagues.

In isolation, deontology is self-limiting as an ethical theory as it focuses specifically on the moral worth of actions rather than consideration of wider factors, such as the outcomes produced by them or the motivation of the moral agent. A strict deontologist would hold that a duty of honesty is fundamental to morality, but this would be to miss taking into account some of the nuances of situations, such as when stating the truth may have negative consequences. Traditional deontology also places an emphasis on duty relating to us as rational beings, using our reason and logic, so leads to debates over complex topics such as abortion where there is disagreement on the status of a foetus and the right to life.

In practice, ODPs can consider deontology in relation to the underpinning principles found in the various codes of conduct that are followed. Aspects such as honesty are core components of professional practice. However, as the next theory demonstrates, nuances do exist that need to be considered with regard to the outcomes of our actions.

Consequentialism

'Consequentialism' (or 'teleological ethics' as it is sometimes called) is concerned more with the consequences or outcomes of an action than with the deed itself. Although different types of consequentialist theories exist, a utilitarian approach is the version most commonly referred to in relation to healthcare ethics.

The main philosophers who developed the utilitarian approach were Jeremy Bentham (1748–1832) and John Stuart Mill (1806–73). Utilitarianism considers an action as morally right if its outcome or consequences are good for the greatest number in society (Mill [1867] 1962). The theory tends to disregard individual rights and considers the well-being of the greatest number to be the most important factor.

In the healthcare context, utilitarianism becomes evident in discussions about the allocation of resources. With only a finite amount of money to spend on healthcare, decisions on where and how it should be spent is a challenge. On a micro level, ODPs will be aware of the day-to-day allocation of resources such as equipment and disposables. However, the macro-level decisions of the organization of healthcare are usually utilitarian, focused on where there is the greatest need in a demographic area. A good example of this was during the COVID-19 pandemic, which saw ICU admissions rise above capacity, leading to shortages of equipment such as ventilators. To navigate this complex ethical dilemma, the British Medical Association (BMA) set out guidance that referred to using utilitarian principles if required (BMA 2022). This approach aims to maximize utility (available resources) with respect to distributive justice (for the greater good) and this could be used generally as a guiding principle for ethical decision-making.

However, utilitarianism is limited in that it considers the general moral outcomes only, so disregards other significant factors. An action is taken to be morally correct if the consequences are beneficial for the majority. It would, therefore, be possible for acts to be endorsed that are contrary to the rights of an individual. For example, if an ODP felt that they needed to breach their duty of confidentiality for a matter regarding a patient, the practitioner would need to weigh up the consequences of the action. The ODP may think that the breach has perceived benefits to others but to the individual patient it could be viewed as a betrayal of trust. Consequences in any given situation are often difficult to predict. An action may have good intentions behind it and have a high probability of there being a good result. In many situations that involve a number of people and options, however, it becomes more difficult to establish which action will produce the best outcome or consequence.

The theories presented in this section have been included to give practitioners a brief overview of different approaches and further reading is both encouraged and recommended to gain greater insight into the history and a more detailed account of each theory.

Stop and think

Take a look at the following scenario and then discuss the ethical aspects involved in relation to the theories that have been outlined in this section.

Imagine that an ODP attends to someone in the street who was having a cardiac arrest and resuscitates them successfully. Due to foreseen but unintended circumstances while undertaking the resuscitation, the ODP has cracked several ribs and badly bruised the person's chest, which results in some long-term problems for the person's recovery.

Using the approaches described for each of the three ethical theories to discuss and debate the points raised by this brief scenario will enable you to deepen your understanding of how the theories relate to contexts you come across in your role as an ODP.

Additional approaches to ethics

In addition to the three theories of Western moral philosophy described so far in this chapter, there are other approaches to exploring ethics in healthcare that can provide insights into the key issues which arise when there are ethical dilemmas.

These approaches can also provide ODPs with a better understanding of the general principles and values that underpin their practice. One of these approaches will now be explored.

The four principles approach

This has become the most popular approach in healthcare ethics and the principles provide useful insights into problem-solving.

The approach is based on a set of principles developed by Thomas Beauchamp (b. 1939) and James Childress (b. 1940) in the early 1980s in the first edition of their book entitled *Principles of Biomedical Ethics*, in which they state that the cluster of four principles does not constitute a general moral theory (Beauchamp and Childress 2019: 14). They then provide a framework for identifying and reflecting on moral problems.

A 'principle' is an essential norm in a system of thought or beliefs, forming a basis of moral reasoning in that system. The 'four principles' concerned here are written in broad terms to widen their scope so they can be applied to all people in any situation. However, principle-based approaches usually infer ethical reasoning and decision-making as parts of a rational process of applying those principles.

The 'four principles' identified by Beauchamp and Childress are as follows.

1 **Autonomy:** This principle is a primary consideration for patient-centred care. It promotes the ability of the person to be independent and self-determining and to make a reasoned choice on the basis of information. It is a highly significant principle in healthcare as it implies that patients have the right not to be constrained, coerced or impeded in any way. It requires respect for each person and for ODPs to promote, not obstruct, their patients' autonomy. However, where this may not be possible, ODPs should follow the principle of beneficence.
2 **Beneficence:** This principle considers the balance of treatment against the risks and costs to the patients. Therefore, ODPs should always act in a way that benefits patients, although it may be that the extent to which ODPs are able to do this is constrained by resources and time.
3 **Non-maleficence:** All treatments involve some harm, even if it is minimal, but the harm should not be disproportionate to the benefits of the treatment. For example, intubation may result in a sore throat (harm), but that is outweighed by the need to secure a patient's airway and ventilate them. Non-maleficence requires ODPs to refrain from doing harm or prevent any action that could cause harm. The premises for this and the previous principle should not be confused: beneficence is about being active in doing good; non-maleficence is about actively preventing harm.
4 **Justice:** This principle is based on fairness and rights, ensuring equality for all. Equality for all in receiving treatment and access to services is notional, as, in practice, it is mainly a case of treating people as individuals and recognizing their differences and needs. For ODPs, this principle takes the form of ensuring that they make the best use of resources allocated and available to them within the confines set, and planning and providing care irrespective of patients' socio-economic status, race, gender or religion. While ODPs may not have the power or ability to control access to and the distribution of resources, they do

have a duty of care and they are responsible for informing the appropriate people of any shortfalls and following these up.

Stop and think

Ethical dilemmas commonly occur in multidisciplinary teams when there are competing moral interests regarding a patient's plan of care. Conflict between acts and omissions when it comes to patient care in the perioperative environment can be complex and may include ethical issues, disagreements in terms of opinions and have legal ramifications.

The four principles approach is a good way to examine such situations. Consider the following situation.

During the laparoscopic treatment of endometriosis, the surgeon notes that the patient's appendix looks acutely inflamed. The patient is under general anaesthesia and consented for laparoscopy +/- procedures relative to the initial diagnosis. The surgeon argues that an appendectomy should be undertaken to prevent the need for a further invasive procedure. However, the anaesthetist insists the consent that has been given is not appropriate for this extra procedure and treatment with antibiotics may be sufficient, given that there were no adverse symptoms reported previously to indicate appendicitis.

Here, an ethical dilemma presents itself against both wider legal issues and team conflict. Arguably, undertaking the appendectomy could be viewed as promoting non-maleficence as the surgeon foresees the additional risk posed by a further invasive procedure. However, if the anaesthetist is correct, then it would promote beneficence to not undertake the additional surgery and prescribe a non-invasive treatment instead.

This issue is further compounded by the consideration of autonomy, as the patient is currently unable to communicate, meaning that the decision will need to be based on considerations of advocacy. Justice has a two-fold application here as the patient is entitled to receive treatment available to them, but also has a right to choose and may favour opting for a less invasive option initially. Further, the extra surgery would have an impact on the wider distribution of time and resources and, therefore, distributive justice on a macro level.

By applying the four principles approach to this example, it is possible to begin to unpick the pertinent ethical issues to arrive at a justifiable decision. This type of decision-making can be enhanced further by using a more structured framework, which is introduced later in this chapter.

Ethics in practice

The theories and guiding standards of our professional values form the structure for our general professional behaviour, but there are many other factors that conflict and create ethical dilemmas. Clinical practice is complex and practitioners have an important role to play in maintaining values and advocating for patients. On a day-to-day basis, ODPs must carefully consider interventions with respect to cultural differences, equality, diversity and inclusivity (HCPC 2023).

To help with this, in the first part of this section, we introduce the importance of values and of advocacy. In the second part, we look at a range of key areas that may present ethical issues with regard to patient care. As you work through this information, you will find it helpful to explore and reflect on real-life situations where ODPs may face difficult and complex dilemmas to see how these ideas would play out in your practice. This will help your professional development regarding the ethical aspects of your practice.

Values

Values play a significant role in the codes of professional practice we follow. Henry et al. (1995: 123) stated that 'the stronger the ethos is in ethical values within a culture of an institution, the more distinctive the institution will be'. It is important to explore values and codes of professional practice as these are fundamental to the relationships in teams. The guiding standards for ODPs can be found in the codes of professional practice, but first it is important to understand what values are.

Both personal and professional values exist. You may share your personal values with family, friends or other social groups, who may have values particular to you. Values emerge from your background, experiences and sense of self. Many values stay constant in your life, while others change and develop over time. Values are often about ideals and there is an element of compromise and change that takes place. These changes can take place as a result of reflection, experience or pressure to align with the values of others in a social context, for example.

Professional values are ones held by those in that profession and maintained by governing or related organizations. The professional values for ODPs are set out by the Health and Care Professions Council (HCPC) in its 'Standards of conduct, performance and ethics' (HCPC 2016). These standards are written in such a way that they are able to be interpreted by all those professional groups regulated by the HCPC. Professional values exist to ensure that the delivery of care meets certain ethical standards and is fair, treats people equally and is non-discriminatory. For ODPs, those values are then further exemplified in the more specific 'Standards of proficiency: Operating Department Practitioners' (HCPC 2023).

Although there are many professions working collaboratively in the perioperative environment that have their own codes and standards, all of them are underpinned by similar core values, such as:

- respecting individual patients;
- obtaining informed consent before any treatment or care is undertaken;
- protecting any confidential information;
- co-operating with others on a team;
- maintaining professional knowledge and competence;
- being trustworthy;
- acting in a way that minimizes or identifies any risk to patients.

The NHS also provides clear values that set out how professionals working in the organization should behave and the approach they should take. The Department of Health (DH) produced 'The handbook to the NHS Constitution for England' (DH 2021), which sets out six values that provide common ground for co-operation so that shared aspirations for the public, patients and members of staff can be achieved. These values are also reflected in recruitment processes, to prevent the kinds of complex issues that can arise when a particular individual's own values conflict with those of their employing institution.

The independent sector has similar guidance for shared values and, in the main, they are not too dissimilar from those of the NHS. Both sectors' values correlate with the six values of the NHS's professional codes and guidance, and encourage a participative level of engagement on the part of patients. But the aspiration of the NHS's values – to respect the rights of patients to be more participative – means that patients need to be not only informed but also have the confidence to engage as much as possible with what is happening regarding their treatment. ODPs should recognize, however, that not all patients want to be fully engaged when they come in to an operating theatre as, often, they would rather not know what is about to happen to them. Their individual needs and wishes should be respected, while at the same time maintaining communication so that they feel they can ask about their care at any time. ODPs need to recognize that, in the perioperative environment, participation can be limited, due to the context in which the care is being delivered.

The value of veracity (truthfulness) is a good example to explore here relative to perioperative care, as it is about telling the truth and preserving honesty, to build trust in the relationship with the healthcare practitioner. Practitioners need to inform patients about the care that they will receive and what they say must be truthful, while remembering that ODPs should only discuss information that is within their scope of practice. Patients rely on practitioners being honest so that they can make rational decisions and act autonomously. However, if a patient were to ask an ODP in the anaesthetic room, 'Can you tell if I will have a painful jaw after the operation as a number of my friends have suffered this and no one has mentioned it to me?' the ODP may choose to refrain from answering this question in a straightforward manner. Instead, they may inform the patient that they are unaware of this, even though there has been a high incidence of this lately, so as not to cause the patient undue anxiety. The ODP would then bear the responsibility for passing the patient's concerns on to the anaesthetist prior to induction so that they can be discussed appropriately with the patient. The patient may need to be prompted by the ODP to ask the anaesthetist to discuss the matter that concerns them as, too often, they feel that they do not want to make a fuss. The matter will need to be handled sensitively and some information may be withheld at this point, as it may be felt insensitive at that stage of the proceedings and may not be of benefit to the patient.

Advocacy

In healthcare, it is important that patients feel supported and able to express their wishes, and this is where the role of advocacy comes in. 'Advocacy' is about supporting an individual or group to enable them to express their views or repre-senting these on their behalf. In practice, it is part of a continuum that may vary depending on the healthcare environment.

In the perioperative environment, patients often feel vulnerable, but the expecta-tion is that professionals will act in their best interests. The role of advocacy in that environment is different from elsewhere in healthcare as there is not much time to build a relationship prior to the start of the care intervention. There are several characteristics that can be drawn from the literature, but it still does not include a clear description of the role of advocacy in the perioperative environment. There are, however, four characteristics that fit well with the role and they include:

- informing patients and promoting informed consent;
- empowering patients and protecting their autonomy;
- protecting the rights and interests of patients when they cannot protect them themselves;
- ensuring that patients have fair access to available resources.

These are not contentious and so are often seen as part of the overall way to be professional in this and other related environments. However, multidisciplinary working involves complex interactions between different professionals and so it is necessary to ensure that everyone is working for a common purpose. In good practice, this is often achieved by holding briefing and debriefing sessions.

The crucial time when a patient requires advocacy is if they are confused and frightened, incompetent or unconscious. It is therefore paramount that ODPs real-ize that fulfilling this role is not about speaking up and representing their views, which are often unknown, but should be about protecting the rights and interests of patients who cannot protect them themselves. It is about ensuring that patients have a clear understanding of their care and are enabled to consult with others, expressing their wishes as appropriate, thereby protecting their autonomy while ensuring that they receive adequate resources to meet their needs.

These factors can cause tension when patients' desires are not conducive to the safe delivery of care, such as wanting to get off the bed or trolley. Insufficient resources can also cause undue tension. Practitioners need to ensure that these requirements or shortfalls are communicated effectively in the organization, especially to those who have responsibility for the wider remit of quality and governance regarding the care delivered.

It needs to be made clear that representing the patient's wishes is the best way to protect and maintain their integrity and, therefore, their autonomy. This is not performing advocacy as if it were a role but acting as a professional who is committed to their duty of care and adhering to their professional standards. If professionals portray what *they* perceive to be the patient's wishes, however well intended, they need to be aware that they may be acting in a paternalistic manner that could be interpreted as being coercive.

Some ODPs working in advanced practice may have longer-term relationships with patients than is usually the case, which means that the idea and approach of the advocacy role will change as the relationship develops. Complying with the regulatory body's requirements and the patient's wishes is still paramount. As for other healthcare professionals, there may be times when your own professional judgement and a patient's views and wishes will not be in harmony. Whatever the case, advocacy must always mean that you protect and are a representative of the patient's needs and values. It is the responsibility of all practitioners to work within the parameters and scope of their practice, including any further education and training required to develop their understanding and to benefit their patients.

Resuscitation

'Resuscitation' means reviving a person by processes aimed at sustaining the functioning of the vital systems, such as the respiratory and cardiac systems, and correcting the acid-base balance. Often this takes place in an emergency situation and little time is given or available for discussion as to whether the person wants to be resuscitated or not. All patients have a right to refuse treatment or resuscitation but unless there has been clear briefing conveying this request, ODPs will be unaware of these wishes. It is important, therefore, that if patients have such wishes, they are made clear to all who are caring for them. There are situations that may override this, mainly due to timings and circumstances. For example, if a patient expresses a wish that 'in the event of my heart stopping, I do not wish to be resuscitated', the kinds of situations that would apply to are extremely difficult and, in practice, practitioners and their colleagues will always act in the patient's best interests.

Do not attempt cardiopulmonary resuscitation (DNACPR) decision

A DNACPR decision will often be drawn up and placed in a patient's notes with their consent form. There are some very good guidelines for decisions relating to cardiopulmonary resuscitation (CPR) by the British Medical Association, Resuscitation Council (UK) and Royal College of Nursing (RCN) (2016) combined, although each hospital will have its own protocols that ODPs will need to have familiarized themselves with and understand. As an ODP it is useful to be aware of the guidance so that you can better understand the process of supporting patients who have a DNACPR decision in place. The NHS uses a process known as 'recommended summary plan for emergency care and treatment', or, ReSPECT (Resuscitation Council UK n.d.), the aim of which is to facilitate a patient-centred approach to DNACPR decisions and how plans are put in place.

A DNACPR decision should always be drawn up in advance of any treatment, following discussion with the patient and/or other family members and/or significant others. This empowers the patient and gives them autonomy in exercising their right to choose how they would like to be treated when they would be least able to do so for themselves.

Such a situation can become complicated if a patient states that they *do* wish to be resuscitated, even when it is explained that to do so could result in the outcome being poor, should they survive. However, doctors do have the right to refuse to treat a patient if they feel that doing so would be both futile and burdensome (Schwartz et al. 2002). Unfortunately, there have been cases where a DNACPR decision was placed in a patient's notes by a medical practitioner but it was not discussed with the patients or others, and this led to relatives questioning the care interventions and being upset.

Refusal of blood

No two ethical issues are the same, as patients are individuals, their conditions and how these can change may be unexpected or happen very quickly, and this is especially true in an operating theatre.

It is usually possible to adjust the planned care for patients who are Jehovah Witnesses to avoid the need for a blood transfusion, which is against their beliefs. However, in an emergency situation, if the need for a transfusion arises due to complications, a patient's decision to refuse a life-saving blood transfusion may cause conflict in the practitioners looking after that patient, who must do good (beneficence) and cause no harm (non-maleficence), yet respect the autonomy of the patient and uphold their right to choose to refuse treatment. The values of the healthcare team and the patient in such a situation may be incongruent, but the patient has a right to refuse even life-saving treatment.

When it comes to parents making this choice for their child in such circumstances, clinicians can seek a court decision to make the child a temporary ward of the court, removing the rights of the parents to withhold consent to a blood transfusion. This is a long process, however, and one that has an impact on the relationship between the parents, the doctor and the healthcare team. Consideration needs to be given to the implications and effects of such a decision and the long-term impacts on the child and their family.

According to Veatch (2000), treating a patient when that treatment has been refused violates their right to make such a self-sacrificing choice as an expression of what they believe in or a particular community they belong to.

From this discussion it is clear that ODPs should be familiar with the issues involved and a good place to start is the guidance on this subject available from the Association of Anaesthetists (2018).

Stop and think

Before moving on, it would be useful to reflect on your own beliefs and ideas in relation to your practice. Also ask yourself the following questions.

- What are the agreed standards of ethical practice in the perioperative environment?
- What role does an ODP play in ethical practice in the team?
- What are the two most frequent ethical dilemmas you experience in your working practice?

Ethical decision-making

It is invaluable to their practice for ODPs to think through issues and problems, especially when they involve an ethical element. If these situations are rehearsed, either by thinking of a scenario or reflecting on a 'real' situation, this can contribute to developing your ability to think about and handle ethical questions in practice.

Structuring this thinking by using a framework of questions can be beneficial, so one such framework is provided later in this section. Using the theories and approaches discussed earlier in this chapter can also support discussion and offer support when resolving conflicts in the professional environment. There are not necessarily any right answers to ethical dilemmas, but ethically sensitive ODPs should apply critical reasoning to making, or contributing to, a judgement or decision – an approach that is reflected in the 'Standards of proficiency' (HCPC 2023).

To recap discussions earlier in this chapter, an ethical dilemma occurs when we are forced to choose between two or more different actions that involve competing moral ideals. Situations that constitute ethical dilemmas are not readily resolved and require careful critical reasoning, as there may be conflict between values and principles, and there may be multiple people involved. Choosing one action may mean that another good is sacrificed.

To take an example, say you promised your friend that you would attend her oncology appointment with her, but on the day you are meant to go, you receive a call from your mother, who has had a serious accident and is on her way to hospital. This dilemma may seem easy – you would go to your mother in the hospital. However, you may be torn between your obligations to your friend, and her life-threatening problem, and your mother. Various factors may influence your thinking. Do you not get along with your mother or can you break your promise to attend the hospital with your friend?

The situation facing you in this scenario is about making a choice between keeping a promise (a moral good) and attending to the care of your mother in hospital (a moral good). In cases such as this that are a personal choice, we can usually simply think about the issue, weigh up the goods and the potential harm each option may present, and can make a decision relatively easily. We do not have to stop and think too much; we go with our gut instinct. In professional practice, however, in the ethical decisions we make, we are accountable to many others and the impacts of those decisions can be far-reaching, so we need to think through the issues to make the best choices possible.

Stop and think

Before moving on to consider the framework of questions, take a moment for a recap of the ethical theories presented earlier in this chapter and begin to think about how they can be applied to the following dilemma.

During the COVID-19 pandemic, healthcare practitioners had to make all kinds of difficult decisions regarding personal moral beliefs. As part of the measures put in place during the pandemic, the UK government introduced a mandate for front-line workers to be fully vaccinated against COVID-19. This mandate led to a debate about the ethical implications of mandatory vaccination. Some of the key issues related to limited research data, long-term outcome monitoring, practitioner autonomy, duty of care and staffing concerns.

The facts, ethics, policy, action (FEPA) framework for ODPs

Developing sound ethical decision-making requires compassion, moral sensitivity and awareness of ethical theories. To develop ethical decision-making skills it can be useful to reflect on previous dilemmas. By using this approach you can look at the ethical aspects of a decision, weighing up the significance of any actions and the impacts they have had on practice. The more complex the situation, the more you need to rely on discussion and dialogue with others about the dilemma, therefore reflection on the problem, supported by the insights and different perspectives of others, will provide all with valuable learning.

To support ODPs, as mentioned, a framework of questions has been developed and included here to guide ethical decision-making. The framework has been informed by a range of existing ethical decision-making models in the literature but is positioned, primarily, in the context of an ODP in a perioperative environment, although it can also be applied to any clinical area. Other models include wider considerations or more steps, but the framework presented here has deliberately been kept as straightforward as possible to make it easy to use while still improving your skills.

Developing your ability to use the framework can support your own growth and your team's handling of such situations. When practised regularly, the method becomes so familiar that it can be worked through without having to refer to all the questions separately.

Examining a moral dilemma requires a logical approach, so framing your critical thinking with a series of questions can guide you towards a decision. The FEPA framework (see Figure 9.1) does both these things so is a useful way to approach such situations. It involves, first, establishing any facts and contextual information available. Next, identifying the ethical issues and consulting ethical theories to obtain perspective. Once the facts and ethical perspectives have been established, the dilemma can then be framed in the context of relevant policies or procedures. Available actions and any remaining questions can then be established. Once a decision has been made, a plan for communicating this should also be made. Making notes and documenting your thought process and timeline is advisable as these help to clarify and justify your course of action.

The FEPA framework uses the following questions (also shown in Figure 9.1) to take you through these steps.

- Do you have all the facts about the situation? Does the situation involve patients and/or others?
- Which members of the team are involved and affected? In what ways are they affected and are there any conflicts?
- What are the ethical issues? Be specific – do they relate to the HCPC's standards, have other professional codes been breached or are there organizational aspects that are of concern?
- What are the specific principles that are of concern? Is this related to professional behaviour, competence, due care, integrity, confidentiality or something else?
- What perspectives do the differing ethical theories present and do they help to articulate the issues with more clarity?

- Do you have all the facts about the situation?
- Does the situation involve patients and/or others?
- Which members of the team are involved and affected? In what ways are they affected and are there any conflicts?

- What are the ethical issues? Be specific – do they relate to the HCPC's standards, have other professional codes been breached or are there organizational aspects that are of concern?
- What are the specific principles that are of concern? Is this related to professional behaviour, competence, due care, integrity, confidentiality or something else?
- What perspectives do the differing ethical theories present and do they help to articulate the issues with more clarity?

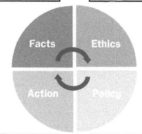

- Based on analysis of the situation, what are the remaining options for action?
- Do you require any further facts or contextual information before being able to make a decision?
- What is your plan with regard to initiating action and how will you communicate this to those involved?

- Are there any internal procedures you need to consider, such as policies or the need to escalate to senior members of staff? Is a whistle-blowing policy involved and/or raising and escalating concerns?
- Consideration needs to be given to organizational guidelines and processes, legal and regulatory aspects, and consequences of the issue. Has this been a long-term problem?

Figure 9.1 The FEPA framework for ODPs

- Are there any internal procedures you need to consider, such as policies or the need to escalate to senior members of staff? Is a whistle-blowing policy involved and/or raising and escalating concerns?
- Consideration needs to be given to organizational guidelines and processes, legal and regulatory aspects, and consequences of the issue. Has this been a long-term issue?
- Based on analysis of the situation, what are the remaining options for action?
- Do you require any further facts or contextual information before being able to make a decision?
- What is your plan with regard to initiating action and how will you communicate this to those involved?

Although it appears formal, the purpose of the framework is to create a logical process. By doing this, working through it brings a sense of order to the issue being examined and it provides a sequence that can contribute towards developing ethical practice.

Practitioners face ethical situations at all stages of their careers, so early engagement with such a model is encouraged. No two situations are exactly the same. To develop towards mastery of the approach requires ODPs to be deliberate about using the framework for debriefs of situations arising in their practice, while they are happening or afterwards, and case scenarios at any time to support them with their recall and reflection on the given ethical dimensions of a situation. Frameworks for ethical decision-making also help us to communicate and you will find that, having analysed a situation using the framework, it will be easier to discuss the issues with others and hear their perspectives, using the framework as a common language.

When working through the ethical decision-making process, either retrospectively as a reflective task or in the moment, it is strongly advised that you also use the help and guidance of those in the team around you, as this will be helpful to you as an individual and the team as you work together.

Stop and think

Think about an ethical dilemma you, or your team, have faced. Work through the FEPA decision-making framework, applying it to aid your critical reflection on the situation and the decision that was made at the time. You may wish to write a formal reflection for this.

If you cannot think of a recent example, consider using the scenario given in the second 'Stop and think' box earlier in this chapter, about a patient undergoing a laparoscopy. Applying the framework will help you to bring together the principles concerned and look at these alongside relevant theories of ethics.

Consider the following questions.

- Was the response based on a clear framework of decision-making?
- If faced with the same dilemma, would your decision be the same, based on the material presented in this chapter?

Conclusion

In this chapter we have only been able to give you an initial insight into this vast subject, so wider reading is highly recommended. It is paramount that ODPs understand the impact the ethical dimension has on their practice and, when working alongside other professionals, they must not be passive participants in the delivery of ethical practice. ODPs are essential members of their teams, with roles and responsibilities both in and outside the perioperative environment, and this gives rise to the need for clarity and a broad understanding of ethics in their practice. Furthermore, with leadership skills being explicitly recognized in the 'Standards of proficiency' (HCPC 2023), it is likely that more ODPs will be undertaking roles in which responsibility for decision-making is central. The HCPC provides a standard outline of how ODPs are required to behave, but a greater understanding of ethical theories, approaches and values allied to these codes will help ODPs to develop further to become ethically sensitive practitioners and moral agents in their practice.

It is fair to say that all professionals involved in the delivery of care in a perioperative environment must collaborate with one another if they are to benefit both patients and the wider health community in a manner that respects the ethical principles of professionalism and healthcare. Healthcare organizations, too, have an obligation to establish processes that identify new procedures or practices which can be seen to be of benefit to patients. However, only with the co-operation of all the healthcare teams can the system produce optimal outcomes and value for individual patients.

It is recommended that you now take forward your learning from this chapter in a number of ways. Reading widely concerning the theories covered here and others is important for deepening your understanding and assisting you in applying the theory to your practice. The further reading and reference section for this chapter is a good starting point for doing this. You are also recommended to reflect on different ethical dilemmas that you have experienced in your clinical practice, using the FEPA decision-making framework to evaluate the ethical dimensions. By consistently evaluating examples over time, you will find that working through complex ethical dilemmas becomes a more fluid and intuitive process. Speaking about your experiences and discussing the ethical considerations with other members of your team who were involved, via debrief, is also an effective way to develop your skills.

Key points

- How ethical theories guide current practice.
- Using a framework to deal with ethical dilemmas.
- What it means to be an ethical practitioner.
- An understanding of personal and professional values.
- Ethics as part of practitioners' practice.

References and further reading

Association of Anaesthetists (2018) Anaesthesia and peri-operative care for Jehovah's Witnesses and patients who refuse blood. London: Association of Anaesthetists. Available at: https://anaesthetists.org/Home/Resources-publications/Guidelines/Anaesthesia-and-peri-operative-care-for-Jehovahs-Witnesses-and-patients-who-refuse-blood (accessed October 2022).

Beauchamp, T.L. and Childress, J.F. (2019) *Principles of Biomedical Ethics*, 8th edn. Oxford: Oxford University Press.

British Medical Association (BMA) (2022) COVID-19: Ethical issues and decision-making when demand for life-saving treatment is at capacity. London: BMA.

British Medical Association (BMA), Resuscitation Council (UK) and Royal College of Nursing (RCN) (2016) Decisions relating to cardiopulmonary resuscitation, 3rd edn, 1st revd. London: BMA, Resuscitation Council (UK) and RCN. Available at: www.resus.org.uk/sites/default/files/2020-05/20160123%20Decisions%20Relating%20to%20CPR%20-%202016.pdf (accessed October 2022).

Department of Health (DH) (2021) The handbook to the NHS Constitution for England. London: DH. Available at: www.gov.uk/government/publications/supplements-to-the-nhs-constitution-for-england/the-handbook-to-the-nhs-constitution-for-england (accessed October 2022).

Health and Care Professions Council (HCPC) (2016) Standards of conduct, performance and ethics. London: HCPC.

Health and Care Professions Council (HCPC) (2023) Standards of proficiency: Operating Department Practitioners. London: HCPC.

Henry, C., Drew, J., Anwar, et al. (1995) The EVA project: University of Central Lancashire, in C. Henry (ed.), *Professional Ethics and Organisational Change in Education and Healthcare*. London: Edward Arnold.

van Hooft, S. (2006) *Understanding Virtue Ethics*. Chesham: Acumen.

Kant, I. ([1785] 1964) *Groundwork of the Metaphysics of Morals*. New York: Harper & Row.

Mill, J.S. ([1867] 1962) *Utilitarianism*. London: Collins.

Newham, R.A. and Hawley, G. (2007) The relationship of ethics to philosophy, in G. Hawley (ed.), *Ethics in Clinical Practice: An Interprofessional Approach*. Abingdon: Routledge.

Resuscitation Council UK (n.d.) ReSPECT. London: Resuscitation Council (UK). Available at: www.resus.org.uk/respect (accessed October 2022).

Schwartz, L., Preece, P.E. and Hendry, R.A. (2002) *Medical Ethics: A Case-Based Approach*. Maryland Heights, MO: W.B. Saunders.

Veatch, R. (2000) Dr does not know best: Why in the new century physicians must stop trying to benefit the patient, *Journal of Medicine and Philosophy*, 25(6): 701–72.

10 Leadership and management for Operating Department Practitioners

Michael Donnellon

Key topics

- Leadership skills
- Management skills
- Theories of change and its management

- Decision-making and problem-solving

Introduction

Leadership and management skills have been identified as essential for all Operating Department Practitioners (ODPs) and other healthcare practitioners, in order to improve services and patient care, and so practitioners have the courage to challenge poor practice (King's Fund 2011). Although there have been many initiatives by many previous governments to develop leadership skills in healthcare, the Mid Staffordshire NHS Foundation Trust public inquiry (Francis 2013), Keogh review (2013) and the report of the Morecambe Bay investigation (Kirkup 2015) have all demonstrated cases when there have been failures in leadership and management in the National Health Service (NHS). The NHS Long Term Plan (2019) identifies that great-quality care needs for there to be great leadership at all levels, and proposes to do more to nurture the next generation of leaders by developing and supporting those with the capability and ambition to reach the most senior levels of the service.

In this chapter, I review the theories of leadership and management, and provide examples of how ODPs can relate these to their practice. You are encouraged to reflect on issues related to leadership and management, but note that there may be no right or wrong answers as, so often, there are many variables to consider.

Why is this relevant?

ODPs practise in a very complex environment where, to deliver safe, effective care to patients, it is necessary to consider many factors, such as staffing levels, equipment and the patients' specific needs. It is not only this process of consideration and an ability to create a synthesis of these factors that is important, however, as

ODPs also need to be able to act on this synthesis by making decisions and then leading or managing the actions that follow. It is therefore essential that, to deliver high-quality patient care, ODPs develop their knowledge of and skills in leadership and management. Leadership is also essential for the continued development of the ODP profession, clinical developments and professional development, if the profession is to be guided successfully through periods of change (College of Operating Department Practitioners (CODP) 2010). Hence, understanding the concept and application of leadership feature in the Health and Care Professions Council's 'Standards of proficiency: Operating Department Practitioners' (HCPC 2023).

Leadership skills

All ODPs will demonstrate skills in leadership throughout their careers, starting while at university by, for example, acting as a group lead when undertaking group work, through to leading a theatre team or maybe, later, managing a department. This demonstrates that these skills underpin the practice of all ODPs, not only those in management roles. If all ODPs demonstrate leadership skills, however, what does that mean?

There are many interpretations of the word 'leadership'. Hersey et al. (2008) define it as a process of influencing the behaviour of either an individual or group, regardless of the reason, in an effort to achieve goals in a given situation. Huczynski and Buchanan (2019) view leadership as the process of influencing the activities of an organized group in its efforts towards setting goals and achieving them. Kotter (2001) thinks of leadership as creating a vision and strategy, communicating and setting a direction, motivating action and aligning people's efforts with that vision.

Stop and think

Using the definitions of leadership and the examples given as a starting point, when have you demonstrated skills of leadership, as a student or registered ODP? How well do you think these definitions apply to your role?

Leadership or management?

It is very common in health and social care to view 'management' and 'leadership' as being broadly the same concept and for these words to be used interchangeably (Martin et al. 2010), but Adair (2008) suggests that there has, and probably always will be, a debate about the overlaps and differences between the two. Current opinion is that they are different concepts, but they do overlap considerably.

In more recent years, the term 'leader' has tended to be used more frequently than 'manager' to describe someone in a professional or medical role who has both management and leadership responsibilities, but there is conflict about these descriptions too. McKimm and Philips (2009) cite Bennis and Nanua (1985), who argue that managers are people who do things right and leaders are people who do the right thing. Barr and Dowding (2009), however, view leaders as being essential to management but the reverse as not being true – that you do not have to be a manager to be a leader, but you do need to be a good leader to be an effec tive manager.

Approaches to leadership

As you might expect, the concept of leadership can mean different things to different people, depending on their perspective. As a result, there is a wide range of leadership theories.

The qualities or traits approach

Popularized in the early part of the twentieth century, this approach – sometimes called the 'great man theory' – assumes that leaders are born, not made. Thus, leadership consists of certain inherited characteristics or personality traits that distinguish leaders from followers – that is, some are born to lead and others are born to be led. Numerous studies have attempted to identify what the qualities and traits of successful leaders are, and their findings have included intelligence, motivation, enthusiasm, initiative, courage, vision, high energy levels, physical appearance, speech, self-confidence, popularity, humour and emotional maturity.

The trait approach has been criticized, however, and Barr and Dowding (2009) suggest that this is because it may negate the part that social class, gender and racial inequalities play in maintaining the status quo for leadership positions. Martin et al. (2010) highlight the conclusion that early trait theory was rejected partly because of the implication that if leadership was only a result of birth, then that would make it the birthright of some privileged people and not others. Adair (2006) argues that the list of qualities or traits is very lengthy and there is a lack of consensus which of them are the key or most important for leadership. Adair (2006) also notes that this approach is ill-suited to being used as a basis for leadership training as it encourages a concentration on selection on the basis of traits that people already have rather than leadership being something that can be taught.

The functional or group approach

In the functional approach, leadership is viewed in terms of how the leader's behaviour affects and is affected by their group of followers (Mullins 2011). Kotter (2001) suggests that by concentrating on the functions fulfilled by a leader, their performance of those functions can be improved by training and, thus, leadership skills can be learned, developed and perfected. Mullins (2011) argues that the way to improve leaders' performance is to, instead, concentrate on the functions that will lead to effective performance by the work group and train leaders to facilitate those.

A contemporary theory on the functional approach to leadership is John Adair's 'action-centred leadership'. A former military lecturer, Adair (2008), argues that a function is what leaders do as opposed to a quality, which is an aspect of what they are. In action-centred leadership, the effectiveness of a leader is dependent on the leader meeting three areas of need in a work group: task needs, team maintenance needs and individual needs. Ideally, the leader should give equal attention to all three areas of need. However, if too much attention is paid to any one particular area of need, this can cause an imbalance, which can interfere with the effectiveness of the group.

Leadership as a behavioural category

In this approach, attention is drawn to the kinds of behaviour people in leadership positions display, including their leadership style. 'Leadership style' is the way in which the functions of leadership are carried out – the way in which a manager typically behaves towards members of the group they are managing. Attention is given to leadership style based on the assumption that subordinates are more likely to work effectively for managers who adopt a certain style of leadership than for managers who adopt other styles (Mullins 2011).

There are many ways to describe leadership styles, including dictatorial, benevolent and charismatic, but the following are prominent among the styles described by writers who put forward this approach.

- **Authoritarian or autocratic style:** The power is held by the leader and they alone exercise control and authority over the group. The leader makes decisions alone and will determine policy and work task goals. Expecting obedience, such a leader will instigate awards and reprimands.
- **Democratic or participative style:** This is a human relations approach – leaders favouring this style ensuring that the focus of power lies more with the group as a whole and that teamwork is encouraged. Members of the group will participate in the decision-making and determining policies and goals.
- **Laissez-faire or genuine style:** There are few established rules, the leader deciding instead to pass the power to the group, allowing its members to work autonomously. However, the leader is available if help is needed. Mullins (2011) highlights that there is sometimes confusion about this style of leadership as the word 'genuine' is to be emphasized rather than the leader who will avoid the trouble spots and not want to get involved.

Stop and think

Are there circumstances in the operating department environment when some styles of leadership are more appropriate than others? For example, during a clinical emergency, which leadership style is most effective?

Contingency leadership theories

Contingency leadership theories hold that there is no single style of leadership that is appropriate in all situations, so focus on the importance of a leader having the necessary flexibility to choose and adapt their approach in response to different situations – that is, having contingencies. One such approach is the path–goal theory, developed by leadership writer Robert House (1996). Path–goal theory is based on the premise that an employee's performance and expectations are greatly affected by the leader's behaviour, as a motivating influence.

Mullins (2011) suggests that in path–goal theory, different types of behaviour can be practised by the same person at different times in varying situations and, by using one of the four styles proposed in the theory, a manager or leader can influence subordinates' perceptions and motivation, smoothing the path to their goals.

Contemporary leadership theories

In addition to the well-documented leadership theories I have mentioned so far, there are some more recent approaches that are referred to as contemporary leadership theories. Gopee and Galloway (2009) suggest that, to an extent, however, these theories represent further developments on earlier leadership theories, taking into account current social, political and organizational factors. Some of the prominent contemporary theories include the following.

- **Charismatic:** In this approach, leadership is based on the personal qualities of the leader, such as their charm, persuasiveness, inspiration and self-confidence.
- **Servant:** American management researcher Robert K. Greenleaf was first to coin the term 'servant leadership', in 1970. In this approach, the servant leader is servant to the team first and leads primarily because of their wish to do good for their followers.
- **Transactional:** Bass and Riggio (2006) write that transactional leadership emphasizes the transaction or exchange that takes place between leaders, colleagues and followers. This exchange is based on the leader discussing with others what is required and specifying the conditions and rewards these others will receive if they fulfil those requirements. The aim in transactional leadership is maintaining equilibrium or the status quo by performing work according to policies and procedures, maximizing self-interest and personal rewards, and emphasizing interpersonal independence (Sullivan 2017).
- **Transformational:** Bass and Riggio (2006) describe transformational leadership as inspiring a team or followers to commit to a shared vision and goals for an organization or unit, challenging them to be innovative problem-solvers, and developing followers' leadership capacity via coaching, mentoring and the provision of both challenge and support. Transformational leaders motivate others to do more than they originally intended and often more than they thought possible. Such leaders tend to have committed and satisfied teams and followers, as they empower them and pay attention to their individual needs and personal development (Bass and Riggio 2006). The transformational leadership approach is favoured by the NHS Leadership Academy, which offers training on the basis that leaders can be developed to 'transform' the behaviour of teams so they can achieve common goals or bring about change.

Stop and think

Looking at the contemporary leadership theories, can you identify if you or any team you have worked in display any of these styles?

Give examples of how a transformational leader can improve teamwork in a perioperative environment.

Leadership and the NHS

Leadership learning in pre-registration programmes

Given that the future NHS workforce must have the right skills, values and behaviour to deliver quality care, Health Education England (HEE 2018) produced a guidance document to enable higher education institutions to deliver leadership development through an evidenced-based framework in pre-registration healthcare curricula. The leadership learning model consists of three stages of developing as a leader in pre-registration (with a focus on stages, working with others, improving healthcare) and three phases of integrating leadership learning into the curricula (such as the principles of programme design, key programme content, key approaches to teaching and learning).

The Council of Deans of Health (Kolyva et al. 2018) has highlighted the importance of teaching leadership experience, as opposed to leadership theory, and how students can be motivated to be leaders from the start of their higher education experience. The Council of Deans of Health has established a student leadership programme that offers innovative ways to develop leadership skills in future healthcare professionals. Targeted at 150 students on nursing, midwifery and Allied Health Professionals (AHP) courses, the programme offers exposure to leadership development through role modelling, reflection, networking and mentoring.

NHS Leadership Academy

The purpose of the NHS Leadership Academy is to help all in the NHS to discover their full leadership potential and for this to have a direct positive impact on patients by raising standards of health and care. It offers a range of tools, models and programmes to support staff, organizations and local partners to develop leaders, celebrating and sharing where outstanding leadership makes a real difference. The NHS Leadership Academy has produced the 'Healthcare Leadership Model', to help those who work in health and care to become better leaders. The model is made up of nine 'leadership dimensions':

1 inspiring shared purpose;
2 leading with care;
3 evaluating information;
4 connecting our service;
5 sharing the vision;
6 engaging the team;
7 holding to account;
8 developing accountability;
9 influencing for result.

As well as the Healthcare Leadership Model, the NHS Leadership Academy has produced a number of programmes that are tailored to help members of staff prepare for leadership, whatever stage they are at in their career. These are applicable to ODPs who are interested in healthcare leadership, whether this will be their first clinical leadership role or they aspire to lead a large department.

Compassionate leadership

A national framework for action to improve and develop leadership in NHS-funded services was published by the National Improvement and Leadership Development Board in 2016 – 'Developing people – improving care'. The framework presents a set of capabilities that are the intended outcomes of this action, one of which is to develop compassionate, inclusive leadership skills for leaders at all levels. Professor Michael West, an expert on leadership in health services and a contributor to the framework, when defining compassionate leadership, explained that it consists of attending, understanding, empathizing and helping (West et al. 2017). Compassionate leaders, therefore, are those who take an interest in (pay attention to) and value their members of staff; they will take time to listen to and respond empathetically to them, alleviating any distress. Compassionate leaders value diversity, too, and they have the ability to share their vision and inspire others to also act with compassion.

The four pillars of practice

Originally associated with advanced clinical practice, the four pillars of practice can also be employed in pre-registration curricula and multiprofessional career frameworks. The four pillars are:

- clinical practice
- leadership and management
- education
- research.

The four pillars can be used at any level of practice and for any job role, though the emphasis on each pillar will vary according to the level and role. For example, the emphasis may be on the clinical practice pillar for a Band 5 ODP, whereas for an ODP who is a theatre manager (typically a Band 8 role), the focus will be more on leadership and management.

Management skills

'Management' is a generic term that is subject to many interpretations. However, at its most basic, it may be viewed as 'making things happen' (Mullins 2011) and so can be regarded as:

- taking place in a structured organization setting with prescribed roles (such as in an NHS trust or independent hospital in the roles of theatre manager, team leader or principle ODP)
- directed towards the attainment of aims and objectives (operating theatre efficiency or management of sickness absence, for example)
- achieved through the efforts of other people (a perioperative multidisciplinary team)
- using systems and procedures (which would include the Department of Health and Social Care or local NHS trust policies).

Theories of management

There have been numerous theories of management published. However, the four main conventional approaches are:

- classical (including scientific management and bureaucratic)
- human relations
- systems
- contingency.

The classical approach

Although one of the earliest management theories, Gopee and Galloway (2009) imply that this approach can still easily be observed in bureaucratic organizations today. In this approach, the emphasis is on improving the organization's structure as a means of increasing efficiency. Attention is given to the division of work and a formal structure is established regarding exactly who does which job, there are clear definitions of duties and responsibilities, and established rules and procedures for various activities. There is an emphasis on a hierarchy of management and formal organizational relationships (Mullins 2011).

Henri Fayol (1841–1925) and Lyndall Urwick (1891–1983), who integrated the ideas of Fayol and those of other early theorists, were two of the main initial developers of this theory of management. However, it is perhaps Frederick Taylor (1856–1915) who is the major contributor, as he wrote about and developed his scientific management approach. Taylor believed that in the same way that there is a best machine for each job, so there is a best method of working to do a job. To discover what that method is, he broke jobs down into discrete tasks to find out the most effective and time efficient way to perform each one. He also believed that each employee's abilities and limitations should be identified, so that workers could be matched to the job most appropriate for their skills, and financial incentives are a motivator for increasing levels of output (Marquis and Huston 2009).

Rees and Porter (2008) identify that, collectively, the classical theorists viewed workers as rational beings who are capable of working to high levels of efficiency, provided they are properly selected, trained, directed, monitored and supported. Although Taylor's work has often been criticized, he has left a legacy of such practices as the study of work, payment by results and production control.

Stop and think

Could the classical approach to management be used effectively to improve efficiency in operating theatres? Make a list of how, in a day surgery setting, tasks could be allocated to different grades of staff according to their training and educational qualifications, experience and competence.

The human relations approach

During the 1920s, theorists began to pay attention to the social factors at work and to the behaviour of employees in organizations. The 'human relations' era had begun and was to emphasize people rather than machines. Leading writers who proposed this approach are Mary Parker Follett (1868–1933) and Rensis Likert (1903–81). Marquis and Huston (2009) note that Follett believed managers should have authority *with* rather than *over* their employees and so solutions could be found that satisfied both the employer and employee without having one side dominate the other.

Studies undertaken by Elton Mayo (1880–1949) at the Hawthorne Works of the Western Electric Company near Chicago between 1927 and 1932 became a landmark development in the human relations approach. Mayo discovered that if managers paid special attention to workers, productivity was likely to increase and this also happened if people worked in groups, especially when the groups were self-selected.

Later developments of the human relations approach are, for example, the neo-human relations theories, which include concepts developed by Abraham Maslow (1908–70, known for his hierarchy of human needs), Frederick Herzberg (1923–2000) and Douglas McGregor (1906–64). McGregor argued that the style of management adopted is a function of the manager's attitudes towards human nature and behaviour at work (Mullins 2011). He labelled this 'Theory X and Theory Y'. 'Theory X' managers assume that their employees are essentially lazy, need constant supervision and direction, show little responsibility and avoid it too. 'Theory Y' managers, however, believe that their employees enjoy their work, are self-motivated, ambitious, problem-solvers and willing to meet the organization's goals.

Gopee and Galloway (2009) argue that the human relations theory is the most appropriate approach for managing healthcare staff, given that the whole ethos of health services is founded on caring and the well-being of people. For example, an ODP manager could take into account an individual member of staff's personal and professional development needs by:

- monitoring how a new member of staff is 'settling in' to the operating department;
- identifying continuing professional development (CPD) opportunities, allowing a member of staff to attend workshops, courses or conferences;
- supporting a member of staff in being creative and encourage them to develop practice improvement projects for the benefit of the department.

The systems approach

The systems approach attempts to consider and reconcile the advantageous aspects of the classical and human relations approaches.

A major contributor to this approach was Ludwig von Bertalanffy (1901–72). Essentially, this approach recognizes organizations as consisting of various systems and subsystems, and directs managers to view their organizations as both a whole and as part of a larger environment (Mullins 2011). Huber (2010) explains that a key principle of the systems theory is that changes in one part of a system affect other parts, creating a ripple in the whole.

The contingency approach

Gopee and Galloway (2009) view the contingency approach as the belief that there is no one optimum state in an organization, so there is no one best and universally applicable management approach, and its success is dependent – or 'contingent' – on the nature of the tasks it is designed to deal with and the nature of environmental influences. There are many variables and situational factors that have an influence on organizational performance.

What do managers do?

Management consultancy is big business and the modern management gurus (Michael Porter, Tom Peters, Peter Drucker, Coimbatore Prahalad and Gary Hamel, to name but a few) have made small fortunes from their publications and talks on how managers can 'gain competitive advantage' for their organizations.

Prior to all this, Henri Fayol, in the early twentieth century, first defined managerial activity as the process of forecasting, planning, organizing, commanding, co-ordinating and controlling (Pettinger 2007). Mullins (2011) highlights five slightly different basic operations in the work of a manager, as identified by Peter Drucker, which are setting objectives, organizing, motivating and communicating, measures and developing people.

Canadian academic and management guru Henry Mintzberg suggested that there are, in fact, ten common roles for managers, which can fall into three categories. Mintzberg (1980) recognized that people who 'manage' have formal authority over the unit they command, which leads to a special position of status in that organization. The roles are given in Table 10.1, with examples that are relevant for ODPs in managerial positions.

Table 10.1 Ten common roles of a manager

Category	Role	Examples for ODPs
Informational	Monitor	Gathers and assesses information related to theatre use, costs and budgets.
	Disseminator	Passes on information to members of staff, such as in a team brief, awareness of the MHRA safety warnings, alerts and recalls.
	Spokesperson	Participates in conferences and meetings outside the organization, such as with the CODP or the partner higher education institute (HEI).
Interpersonal	Figurehead	Represents the department at meetings, such as at directorate, divisional level.
	Leader	Directs and motivates staff and students by influencing – a role model approach.
	Liaison	Networks with people in and outside the organization.
Decisional	Entrepreneur	Initiates change by or as an example.
	Disturbance handler	Deals with disputes between members of staff that arise in the workplace environment
	Resource allocator	Decides where to direct resources (both physical, such as members of staff, and materials, equipment).
	Negotiator	Participates in negotiations in their team, their own organization and external ones, such as with the human resources department and trade unions.

Managing people

Although there are many aspects to management, one essential quality of a successful ODP manager is an ability to manage people effectively. Mullins (2011) argues that people generally respond in a similar way to how they are treated. If you give a little, you will invariably get a lot back. This is particularly relevant in the operating department environment, given that ODPs need to be very flexible about their working hours to cover the unpredictability of operating lists. The majority of employees will respond constructively if they are treated with consideration and respect. So, how does a manager 'manage people' effectively? Mullins (2011) suggests applying philosophies that include the following qualities:

- consideration, trust and respect
- giving recognition and credit
- involvement and availability
- fair and equitable treatment
- positive action on an individual basis
- emphasis on end results
- staff and customer (patient) satisfaction.

Stop and think

In your work environment, do you know a manager who demonstrates any or all the qualities listed under the heading 'Managing people'? How effective do you think they are?

Have you ever experienced an 'unapproachable manager'? What was so 'unapproachable' about them? Was there an element of 'fear' involved? Were there certain 'good' times when you could approach the manager and 'bad' times when you could not?

Ultimately, which managers get the most out of their members of staff?

Management by objectives (MBO)

Peter Drucker (1909–2005) developed and first put forward his MBO model in 1954 and, as Gopec and Galloway (2009) note, it directly affects contemporary management in healthcare. In this style of management, the manager aims to 'juxtapose' the organization's objectives with those of the individual employee and with the employee's development needs. During the annual review meeting, the manager and employee jointly identify objectives and targets that are common to both the employee and organization, together with a standard and measurement of performance.

Theories of change and its management

Change is inevitable in operating department practice and, in particular, in the NHS. There are various reasons for change, including instances when it is:

- initiated by the election of a new government that implements new policies or reforms
- introduced by a review of government policy or a report
- introduced by the outbreak of an illness or disease causing an epidemic or pandemic
- initiated by means of evidence-based practice
- required to meet the needs and expectations of an ageing population
- due to the impact of technological advances in treating disease.

The ways in which people adapt to and adopt new innovations (or change) varies and these different styles have been categorized by Rogers and Shoemaker (1972).

- **Innovators** are eager to try new ideas. They have a desire to be rash, daring, take risks and are willing to accept an occasional setback.
- **Early adopters** accept and apply new ideas early on. It is the early adopters who other individuals see as the 'ones to watch' before using a new idea themselves, so they serve as role models for the other members of the team.
- **Early majority** adopt new ideas before the average members of a team, but still after the early adopters, as they may deliberate for some time before completely embracing a new idea.
- **Later majority** adopt new ideas slightly after the average members of a team, as they approach innovations with a sceptical and cautious air.
- **Laggards** are the last to adopt an innovation, as their decisions are usually made in in line with what has been done in previous generations. The tend to be suspicious of innovations, innovators and change agents.

Although change can bring its positives, poorly introduced or 'unmanaged' change can be perceived by employees as threatening and fraught with difficulties. Thornhill et al. (2000) highlight that the implementation of change is likely to be problematic. This is especially likely to be the case in situations where the type of change involves people, and in which personal relationships and emotional responses are predominant. Likewise, Cameron and Green (2009) argue that the consequences of change are significant. For example, who benefits from the change – the employees or the employer? Who will be the winners and who will be the losers?

Much of the change management literature positions leadership as the key source of energy for change. Carnall (2007) highlights that the process of change can be summarized as involving two elements: leaders and followers. Leaders give signals that changes are needed but without followers, no change is possible because leaders cannot do everything. Not all followers will embrace change and not all followers will resist change.

Stop and think

What has been the main impact of change on your practice?

Reflect on what changes have been made in your workplace since you started working as an ODP. What 'triggered' those changes? Have some changes been reversed?

Is there an aspect of your practice that you consider would benefit from change?

Models of change

Documented in the management literature are numerous models and theories of organizational change, each model having its own potential benefits or weaknesses. Some of the prominent ones you will find are:

- Lewin's three-step model (1947)
- Lippitt's seven-phase model of planned change (1958)
- McKinsey's 7-S model (1978)
- Bullock and Batten's four-phase model of planned change (1985)
- Cummins and Huse's eight-phase model (1989)
- Carnall's change management model (1990)
- Bridges' transition model (1991)
- Kotter's 8-step process for leading change (1995).

Two other models are particularly relevant to healthcare:

- plan, do, study, act (PDSA) cycle (1993)
- NHS Change Model (2018).

As with any model or framework, they are tools that can help to provide a structured approach to implementing change, so it is useful to learn about them. The ones that are most relevant to healthcare and, in particular, the work of ODPs, are described briefly in the rest of this section.

Lewin's three-step model

Kurt Lewin's work dominated the theory and practice of change management for more than 40 years (Burnes 2004a). However, in the past 20 years or so his three-step model has attracted some major criticisms, such as that it is too simplistic for the modern era. Lewin (1890–1947) was a social scientist and had written extensively about a number of approaches to organizational change, including field theory, group dynamics and action research. However, it is his work regarding the three-step model, that is often cited as his key contribution to organizational change.

Lewin argues that a successful change project involves the following three steps (Burnes 2004a).

1 **Unfreezing:** Lewin believed that the stability of human behaviour is based on a quasi-stationary equilibrium supported by a complex field of driving and restarting forces. If the equilibrium is destabilized (unfrozen), old behaviour can be discarded and new behaviour adopted successfully.
2 **Moving:** From less acceptable to more acceptable types of behaviour (change).
3 **Refreezing:** Seeking to stabilize the group at a new point of quasi-stationary equilibrium to ensure that the new types of behaviour are relatively safe from regression. In terms of an organization, refreezing often requires changes to its culture, norms, policies and practices.

Bullock and Batten's four-phase model of planned change

In the early 1980s, R. J. Bullock and Donde Batten developed their integrated model of planned change based on a review and synthesis of more than 30 models of planned change (Burnes 2004a). Its four phases are as follows.

1 **Exploration phase:** An organization explores and decides whether it wants to make specific changes to its operations and, if so, commits resources to planning the changes. A consultant or facilitator is appointed to assist with the planning.
2 **Planning phase:** Forming an understanding of the organization's problems or concerns begins. Information is collected to establish a correct diagnosis of what these are. Change goals are established and key decision-makers are persuaded to approve and support the chosen changes.
3 **Action phase:** The organization implements the changes derived during the planning phase, moving the organization from its current state to the desired future state. Evaluation of the activities implemented takes place and results are fed back so that any necessary adjustments or refinements can be made.
4 **Integration phase:** Consolidating and stabilizing the changes that have been established are the main actions undertaken during this phase, so that the changes that have been implemented become part of the organization's normal everyday operations. Reinforcement of the new behaviour, through feedback and reward systems, is also undertaken during this time.

Kotter's eight-step process for leading change

Acclaimed author and leading authority on leadership and change, John Paul Kotter (b. 1947) presented his eight-step model in his book *Leading change* (1996). Kotter's model first appeared in an article in the March–April 1995 issue of the *Harvard Business Review*. In the article, Kotter lists the mistakes organizations have often made when trying to effect real change and infers that his eight-step change framework makes sense as a roadmap, helping people to talk about transformation, change problems and change strategies.

Plan, do, study, act (PDSA) cycle

The PDSA cycle originates from the work undertaken by Deming in 1950 (Moen and Norman 2010) and is favoured by NHS England and NHS Improvement, and the American Institute for Healthcare Improvement. The cycle can be used to test an idea by temporarily trialling a change and assessing the impact, allowing any refinement of the idea to be worked out prior to its application.

Langley et al. (1994) have since added three questions to supplement the cycle and the combined framework is now called the 'model for improvement'. The questions invite consideration to be given to the aim, how to know if the change is an improvement and what measures of its success will be used, and what changes can be made to result in an improvement. NHS England and NHS Improvement (2021) set out the four stages in this cycle as follows:

• **plan** the change to be tested or implemented
• **do** carry out the test or change
• **study** based on the measurable outcomes agreed before starting out, collect data before and after the change and reflect on the impact of the change and what was learned
• **act** plan the next change cycle or full implementation.

Stop and think

How could the application of the PDSA cycle and model for improvement be used to introduce a quality improvement (QI) initiative to your operating theatre?

NHS Change Model

The NHS Change Model was originally developed in 2012 to support the NHS in adopting a shared approach to leading change and transformation. The model was created by senior leaders, clinicians, commissioners, providers and improvement activists who wanted to become involved in building the energy for change across the NHS by adopting a systematic and sustainable approach to improving quality care (NHS 2018).

The model brings together collective improvement knowledge and experience from across the NHS in the following eight key components:

- spread and adoption;
- improvement tools;
- project and performance management;
- measurement;
- system drivers;
- motivate and mobilize;
- leadership by all.

Resistance to change

Despite the potential positive outcomes, change is often resisted at both individual and organizational levels (Mullins 2011). Carnall (2007) suggests that change is difficult as one must inevitably deal with people issues and an uncertain future. Tyler (2007) identified that a common problem associated with change is that it may create unintended consequences.

Mabey and Salaman (1995, cited in Thornhill et al. 2000) mention a number of perceptions of the management of change that affect reactions to it. Among these factors are whether change is perceived as 'deviant or normal' and 'threatening or desirable'. Change judged as deviant is that which may have been perceived as imposed and outside prevailing cultural norms, so it is likely to generate resistance at various levels. Change seen as threatening is also likely to meet resistance and its implementation will need to be handled carefully if it is to overcome the fear associated with how it has been perceived.

Resistance to change can take two forms: overt, which is when people are open about why they are against the change (the preferable form), or covert, which is when individuals or groups secretly try to sabotage the change. The covert form is therefore much more damaging and harder to deal with than the overt form (Marquis and Huston 2009).

Mullins (2011) identifies common reasons behind individuals' resistance to change. General examples for these reasons are given in Table 10.2, together with ones that ODPs might give in the face of change.

Table 10.2 Reasons for resistance to change

Reasons	Examples	Examples for ODPs
Selective perception	People can have a biased view of a particular situation	Role boundaries affecting view (such as anaesthesia, surgical, post-anaesthetic care)
Habit	Habits serve as a means of comfort and security	Regular shift patterns Being allocated regularly to a particular operating theatre Usual car parking spot!
Inconvenience or loss of freedom	Change could make life more difficult	Changes to regular shift patterns Introduction of some 'clocking on/clocking off' system
Economic implications	Either directly or indirectly, a reduction in pay or other rewards or a threat to job security	Reduction in amount for 'on call' or extra duty payments Pay freeze Review of role or pay banding
Security in the past	When faced with new or unfamiliar ideas or methods, people may reflect on a sense of there being security in the past	Change due to the introduction of a new policy or practice Change due to the introduction of new equipment Change due to working with a new team
Fear of the unknown	Changes in work organization may present a degree of uncertainty leading to anxiety or fear	Restructuring of directorate or department Amalgamation of two NHS trusts

Overcoming resistance to change

Carnall (2007) suggests that much of what is referred to as 'resistance to change' is, in fact, 'resistance to uncertainty', so resistance stems more from how the process is handled and less from what is being changed. If people understand what is to be achieved, why, how and by whom, this will contribute to understanding what is happening and what it will mean for them.

In a prominent article on the subject, Kotter and Schlesinger (1979) argued that many managers underestimate not only the variety of ways in which people can react to change but also the ways in which managers can have a positive influence on specific individuals or groups during change. Kotter and Schlesinger (1979) set out the following approaches as possible solutions to resistance to change.

- **Education and communication:** One of the most commonly used solutions to resistance to change is to educate people about it beforehand. Communication of ideas helps people to see the need for and the logic of change and, once persuaded, people will often then help to implement the change.

- **Participation and involvement:** If the initiators involve the potential resistors in some aspect of the design and implementation of the change, they can often forestall resistance. With a participative change effort, the initiators listen to the people the change involves and incorporate their advice.
- **Facilitation and support:** This process might include providing training in new skills or simply listening and giving emotional support. Facilitation and support are most helpful when fear and anxiety lie at the heart of resistance.
- **Negotiation and agreement:** Offering incentives to active or potential resistors is one way to deal with resistance. Negotiation is particularly appropriate when it is clear that someone is going to lose out as a result of change and yet their power to resist it is significant.
- **Manipulation and co-opting:** Co-opting an individual usually involves giving them a desirable role in the design or implementation of the change. Co-opting a group involves giving one of its leaders or someone it respects a key part to play in the design or implementation of the change.
- **Explicit and implicit coercion:** With this approach, people are forced to accept a change by being explicitly or implicitly threatened (such as with loss of promotion possibilities) or transferred to another department in the organization or dismissed.

Acceptance of change

Kirkpatrick (1993) identified nine reasons for people either accepting or welcoming change, which are that they:

- expect more favourable working conditions or an increase in income and status;
- expect more opportunities for growth, recognition and promotion;
- think the change will provide new challenges and lessen boredom;
- think the change is needed and the timing is right;
- like or respect the person or department introducing the change;
- like the way the change has been introduced;
- contributed to or had some input in the change;
- have positive feelings about the organization or their jobs;
- have been influenced positively towards it by their peers or leaders of their peer groups.

Stop and think

Consider a day surgery unit that currently operates Monday to Friday only. The theatre manager wishes to introduce a rotational system that would also cover weekends, which will require all members of staff to be included.

If you were given responsibility for implementing this change, what should you consider and how would you approach it?

Decision-making and problem-solving

Earlier in this chapter, it was noted that decision-making is part of the manager's role. Huber (2010) suggests that decision-making is the essence of leadership and management, while Marquis and Huston (2009) write that decision-making is often thought to be synonymous with management and is one of the criteria by which management expertise is judged.

Although the terms 'decision-making' and 'problem-solving' appear similar, they are not synonymous. Decision-making may or may not involve a problem, but it does involve selecting one of several alternatives, each of which may be appropriate under the circumstances. Problem-solving, however, involves diagnosing a problem and solving it, which may or may not entail deciding on what the correct solution is (Sullivan and Decker 2009).

Table 10.3 identifies activities encountered by ODPs that require either the making of a decision, identifying a problem and a solution or both.

Decision-making

It can be seen from Table 10.3 that some of the decisions ODPs need to make can be big, some are small and others are either complex or straightforward.

'Routine decisions' are often made by referring to policies and procedures, which can usually produce a satisfactory result in a short period of time.

'Adaptive decisions' are those that need to be made at times when the problem and alternative solutions are somewhat unusual and only partially understood. Such decisions can be arrived at by adapting a decision made in a previous similar situation so it suits this one. There are a number of decision-making techniques or tools that can assist with the problem analysis in these situations, enabling the outcomes for alternative solutions to be compared. These include simple flow charts, decision trees, fishbone diagrams, problem continuums, cause-and-effect diagrams and consequence tables. A 'decision tree' is a graphic model that displays the options, outcomes and risks to be anticipated visually (see Figure 10.1). Normally, decision trees start at the left, identifying the question or problem, and

Table 10.3 Decision-making and problem-solving for activities performed by ODPs

Activities	Decision-making or problem-solving
During the check-in procedure, the patient informs you that they had a drink an hour before their operation	Decision-making
During checking of the anaesthetic machine, a fault is found with the ventilator	Decision-making and problem-solving
During needle, swab and instrument count, a swab is missing	Decision-making and problem-solving
A member of staff phones in sick	Problem-solving
Which member of staff to send on a transfer	Decision-making
A student complains of being unfairly treated by a mentor	Problem-solving

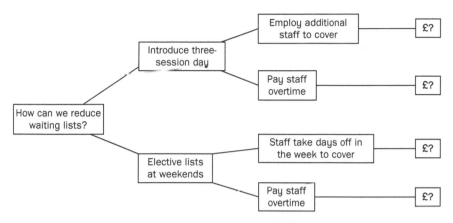

Figure 10.1 Decision tree for the question 'How can we reduce waiting lists?'

flow to the right, identifying the possible options, consequences and costs that become branch nodes. A decision tree may be initiated with a question such as 'How can we reduce waiting lists?'.

There are also 'innovative decisions', which are made when a problem is unusual, unclear or unprecedented, so require that a creative or novel solution is found.

Stott (1992, cited in Barr and Dowding 2009) identified that, in addition, not all decisions are of equal importance and some will involve either a greater or lesser time commitment, some will require additional skills, some will involve many people and some will require greater or lesser levels of resources. In this way, decisions fall into the following main categories.

- **Standard decisions:** Those made on a daily basis, which tend to be repetitive. Solutions are usually found by applying policies or procedures. An example of such a decision is reporting a fault with a piece of equipment to the electro-biomedical engineering (EBME) department.
- **Crisis decisions:** These are made in unexpected situations and require an immediate response with little time to negotiate and plan with others. An example of this kind of decision is being notified that a patient has a ruptured aortic aneurysm and requires immediate surgery.
- **Deep decisions:** Made when there is a requirement for intense planning, reflection and consideration. An example of this type of decision is considering the building of an additional operating theatre or reviewing part of the change management process.

The decision-making process

There are many approaches to decision-making, but here are three that are useful for ODPs to know about.

The 'political decision-making model' is a process in which the particular interests and objectives of powerful stakeholders influence the decisions made by others. For example, clinical commissioning groups, local education and training boards, and regulatory bodies follow this kind of process.

The 'rational decision-making model' is based on making logical, well-grounded, rational choices that maximize the achievement of objectives.

Sullivan and Decker (2009) mention the 'descriptive rationality model', which was developed by Herbert Simon (1916–2001) together with his 'bounded rationality' approach to decision-making in 1955. This model emphasizes the limitations on the rationality of the decision-maker and the situation. It recognizes three ways in which decision-makers depart from the rational decision-making model:

- the decision-maker's search for possible objectives or alternative solutions is limited because of time, energy or money;
- people frequently lack adequate information about problems and cannot control the conditions under which they operate;
- individuals often use a strategy that is not ideal but is good enough under the circumstances to meet the minimum standards of acceptance.

The decision-making process begins when a gap is identified between what is actually happening and what should be happening, and it ends with action that will narrow or close this gap (Sullivan and Decker 2009).

The 'seven-step decision-making model' breaks the process up into individual components. The seven steps are (Sullivan and Decker 2009):

1 identify the purpose;
2 set the criteria;
3 weigh up the criteria;
4 seek alternatives;
5 test alternatives;
6 troubleshoot;
7 evaluate the action.

Whichever model is used, however, care still needs to be taken. Clancy (2003) notes that there is a tendency for managers to unconsciously favour first impressions when making decisions and, once established, a second tendency, known as a 'confirmation bias', can follow. A confirmation bias is the tendency to affirm one's initial impression and preferences when other alternatives are evaluated. Even when decision-making tools are used, therefore, this does not guarantee that a successful, unbiased decision will result, so this is something to be aware of.

Problem-solving

Some problems are self-solving – that is, if the problem runs its natural course, it is solved by those personally involved without the need for any intervention by the manager. However, this can carry a fair amount of risk as the problem can manifest again and when intervention *is* required, the manager may then be faced with a far more complex situation to deal with than was the case with the first instance.

As with decision-making, there are various methods available to solve problems. The simplest is the 'trial-and-error method', which is to apply one solution after another until the problem has been solved or the situation appears to be improving. However, as Huber (2010) infers, managers who use this as their usual strategy for decision-making are seen as ineffective and poor problem-solvers.

The 'experimentation method' is more rigorous than trial and error and can involve the use of pilot projects and trials. An example of this in practice might be the introduction of an on-call system in place of permanent night staff. After a period of time, data could be collected and analysed to determine whether the project has been effective in solving the problem or not.

There are also problem-solving models and one of the most widely used is an equivalent of the seven-step decision-making model – the seven-step problem-solving model. The steps for this model are as follows.

1 **Define the problem:** Does the problem really exist? Is there an existing policy or protocol that could alleviate the problem?
2 **Gather the information:** It is important to gather as much accurate information as possible about the problem from a variety of sources so informed decisions can be made.
3 **Analyse the information:** List and categorize the information.
4 **Develop solutions:** There could be various alternative solutions, so it is important to not only consider the simple solutions but also the more complex ones. Solutions to long-standing problems may have been suggested previously, but take these into account. Past experience may not supply the answer but looking at it can aid the problem-solving process.
5 **Make decision:** After reviewing all the information and identifying possible solutions, select the one that is most applicable and feasible to solve the problem.
6 **Implement the decision:** Implement the preferred solution. Monitor what happens as there is always the risk of unintended consequences materializing.
7 **Evaluate the solution:** After the solution has been implemented, review the plan and compare the results with what was originally the ideal solution.

Marquis and Huston (2009) argue that although this is an effective model, its weakness lies in the amount of time needed to implement it properly.

Stop and think

Looking at the seven-step problem-solving model, how useful would you find this for implementing an effective change in your practice?

You may want to refer back to the 'Stop and think' box below the heading 'Acceptance of change' earlier in this chapter. Looking at the seven steps, how could you apply these to the day surgery scenario?

Group problem-solving

The advantage of groups is that, collectively, they have greater knowledge and experience than any single member and so may produce more solutions or approaches for solving a problem. Together, they can also generate more complete, accurate and less biased information than one person (Sullivan and Decker 2009).

However, Barr and Dowding (2009) argue that some caution must be exercised as individuals may conform to the majority decision, due to group pressure, or feel uncomfortable if they are perceived as an outsider. Also, the leadership of the group is important to how well the problem-solving process works, and this will be influenced by the leader's style, be it autocratic, democratic or laissez-faire.

Conclusion

In this chapter I have examined leadership and management theories and styles, how change can be managed and the complexities of decision-making and problem-solving. Given the ever-increasing demands in and on healthcare services, the NHS requires effective leaders. A key recommendation of the report of the Mid Staffordshire NHS Foundation Trust public inquiry (Francis 2013) identified the particular importance of leaders setting examples of applying the common culture and values of the NHS.

You may recall that at the beginning of this chapter, I stated that leadership and management are essential skills for ODPs and other healthcare practitioners, in order to improve services and patient care. As more and more ODPs are employed in managerial and advance practitioner roles, their leadership and management skills will need to be developed and continue to be as they progress in their careers. Knowledge of these key skills also needs to be included in pre-registration healthcare programmes, as the students of today are the leaders of tomorrow.

Key points

- Leadership skills are increasingly important for ODPs, as is understanding the theories that underpin them.
- Management skills are also key, and knowing about the theories that relate to them.
- Understanding theories of change and its management are essential as ODPs work in a continually changing environment.
- Decision-making and problem-solving are fundamental aspects of the ODP role and there are various approaches that can be used to enable and support these processes.

References and further reading

Adair, J. (2006) *Effective Leadership Development.* London: Chartered Institute of Personnel and Development.

Adair, J. (2008) *The Best of Adair on Leadership And Management.* London: Thorogood Publishing.

Barr, J. and Dowding, L. (2009) *Leadership in Healthcare.* London: Sage.

Bass, B.M. and Riggio, R.E. (2006) *Transformational Leadership*, 2nd edn. Mahwah, NJ: Lawrence Erlbaum.

Burnes, B. (2004a) Kurt Lewin and the planned approach to change, *Journal of Management Studies*, 41(6): 977–1002.

Burnes, B. (2004b) *Managing Change: A Strategic Approach to Organisational Dynamics*. Harlow: Financial Times Prentice Hall.

Cameron, E. and Green, M. (2009) *Making Sense of Change Management*, 2nd edn. London: Kogan Page.

Carnall, C.A. (2007) *Managing Change in Organizations*, 5th edn. Harlow: Financial Times Prentice Hall.

Clancy, T.R. (2003) The art of decision making, *Journal of Nursing Administration*, 33(6): 343–9.

College of Operating Department Practitioners (CODP) (2010) Framing the future role and function of Operating Department Practitioners: Discussion paper. London: CODP.

Francis, R. (2013) Report of the Mid Staffordshire NHS Foundation Trust public inquiry: Executive summary. HC 947. London: The Stationery Office. Available at: https://assets.publishing.service.gov.uk/government/uploads/system/uploads/attachment_data/file/279124/0947.pdf (accessed September 2022).

Gopee, N. and Galloway, J. (2009) *Leadership and Management in Healthcare*. London: Sage.

Health and Care Professions Council (HCPC) (2023) Standards of proficiency: Operating Department Practitioners. London: HCPC.

Health Education England (HEE) (2018) Maximising leadership learning in the pre-registration healthcare curricula. London: HEE.

Hersey, P., Blanchard, K.H. and Johnson, D.E. (2008) *Management of Organizational Behavior: Leading Human Resources*, 9th edn. Upper Saddle River, NJ: Prentice Hall.

House, R.J. (1996) Path–goal theory of leadership: Lessons, legacy, and a reformulated theory, *Leadership Quality*, 7(3): 323–52.

Huber, D. (2010) *Leadership and Nursing Care Management*, 4th edn. Maryland Heights, MO: Saunders Elsevier.

Huczynski, A. and Buchanan, D.D. (2010) *Organizational Behaviour: An Introductory Text*. Harlow: Financial Times Prentice Hall.

Huczynski, A. and Buchanan, D.D. (2019) *Organisational Behaviour*. London: Pearson.

Keogh, B. (2013) Review into the quality of care and treatment provided by 14 hospital trusts in England: Overview report. London: National Health Service. Available at: www.basw.co.uk/system/files/resources/basw_85333-2_0.pdf (accessed September 2022).

King's Fund, The (2011) *The Future of Leadership and Management in the NHS: No More Heroes*. London: The King's Fund.

Kirkpatrick, D.L. (1993) Riding the winds of change, *Training and Development*, 47(2): 28–32.

Kirkup, B. (2015) The report of the Morecambe Bay investigation. London: The Stationery Office. Available at: https://assets.publishing.service.gov.uk/government/uploads/system/uploads/attachment_data/file/408480/47487_MBI_Accessible_v0.1.pdf (accessed September 2022).

Klein, R. (1989) *The Politics of the NHS*. London: Longman.

Kolyva, K., Butt, N. and Eames, J. (2018) #150Leaders: Fostering student leadership. London: Council of Deans of Health.

Kotter, J.P. (1995) Leading change: Why transformation efforts fail, *Harvard Business Review*, May–June. Available at: https://hbr.org/1995/05/leading-change-why-transformation-efforts-fail-2 (accessed September 2022).

Kotter, J.P. (1996) *Leading Change*. Boston, MA: Harvard Business School Press.

Kotter, J.P. (2001) What leaders really do, *Harvard Business Review: The Magazine*, pp. 85–98.

Kotter, J.P. and Schlesinger, L.A. (1979) Choosing strategies for change, *Harvard Business Review*, 57(2): 106–14.

Langley, G., Nolan, K. and Nolan, T. (1994) The foundation of improvement, *Quality Progress*, 27(6): 81–7.

Marquis, B.L. and Huston, C.J. (2009) *Leadership Roles and Management Functions in Nursing: Theory and Application*, 6th edn. Philadelphia, PA: Wolters KluwerHealth/Lippincott Williams & Wilkins.

Martin, V., Charlesworth, J. and Henderson, E. (2010) *Managing in Health and Social Care*, 2nd edn. Abingdon: Routledge.

McKimm, J. and Philips, K. (2009) *Leadership and Management in Integrated Services*. Exeter: Learning Matters.

Mintzberg, H. (1980) *The Nature of Managerial Work*. Englewood Cliffs, NJ: Prentice Hall.

Moen, R.D. and Norman, C.L. (2010) Circling back: Clearing the myths about the Deming cycle and seeing how it keeps evolving quality progress, *Quality Progress*, 43(11): 22–8.

Mullins, L.J. (2011) *Essentials of Organisational Behaviour*, 3rd edn. Harlow: Pearson.

National Health Service (NHS) (2018) The Change Model. London: NHS. Available online at: www.england.nhs.uk/sustainableimprovement/change-model (accessed September 2022).

National Health Service (NHS) (2019) The NHS Long Term Plan. London: NHS. Available at: www.longtermplan.nhs.uk/wp-content/uploads/2019/08/nhs-long-term-plan-version-1.2.pdf (accessed September 2022).

National Improvement and Development Board (2016) Developing people – improving care: A national framework for action on improvement and leadership development in NHS-funded services. London: NHS Improvement. Available at: https://eoe.leadershipacademy.nhs.uk/wp-content/uploads/sites/6/2019/04/10591-NHS_-Improving_Care-Summary.pdf (accessed September 2022).

NHS England and NHS Improvement (2021) Plan, do, study, act (PDSA) cycles and the model for improvement. London: NHS England and NHS Improvement. Available at: www.england.nhs.uk/wp-content/uploads/2022/01/qsir-pdsa-cycles-model-for-improvement.pdf (accessed September 2022).

Pettinger, R. (2007) *Introduction to Management*. Basingstoke: Palgrave Macmillan.

Rees, W.D. and Porter, C. (2008) *Skills of Management*, 6th edn. London: South-Western Cengage Learning.

Rogers, E.M. and Shoemaker, F.F (1972) *Communications of Innovations: A Cross-Cultural Approach*, 2nd edn. New York: Free Press.

Sullivan, E.J. (2017) *Effective Leadership in and Management in Nursing*, 9th edn. London: Pearson.

Sullivan, E.J. and Decker, P.J. (2009) *Effective Leadership and Management in Nursing*, 7th edn. Upper Saddle River, NJ: Prentice Hall.

Thornhill, A., Lewis, P., Millmore, et al. (2000) *Managing Change: A Human Resource Strategy Approach*. Harlow: Financial Times Prentice Hall.

Tyler, S. (2007) *The Manager's Good Study Guide*, 3rd edn. Maidenhead: Open University Press.

West, M., Eckert, R., Collins, B., et al. (2017) *Caring to Change: How Compassionate Leadership Can Stimulate Innovation in Healthcare*. London: The King's Fund.

11 Lifelong learning and continuing professional development for Operating Department Practitioners

Susan Parker

Key topics

- Professionalization and continuing professional development (CPD)
- Why CPD?
- Defining lifelong learning and CPD
- Exploring CPD and its benefits

- Which forms of learning constitute CPD?
- Planning and managing your CPD
- What to do if you are selected to submit your CPD profile

Introduction

The Operating Department Practitioner (ODP) profession has undergone a series of rapid, successive changes – changes that have brought continuing professional development (CPD) to the forefront of our professional practice. Prior to its introduction as a prerequisite for professional regulation, many ODPs may not have been actively engaged in learning beyond what was required to fulfil their immediate roles and practice contexts. In this chapter I explore the concepts and practices of CPD, from defining what CPD is and examining the nature of its relationship to professional practice, to its importance as a measure of our competence when set against an increasingly complex and changing healthcare environment.

Why is this relevant?

Healthcare and the healthcare environment are continually changing, and this is especially apparent in the perioperative environment. Medical care and surgical treatment are advancing rapidly, with the introduction of new technology, innovations, procedures and equipment to treat and manage patients. To remain current and credible when set against these developments in healthcare practices, the role of ODP, led by the College of Operating Department Practitioners (CODP), has itself undergone a series of changes. The introduction of the Diploma of Higher Education (DipHE) in Operating Department Practice in 2001 saw a more academic approach being taken to the education requited to enter the profession, with higher education institutes (HEIs) also becoming the sole providers of courses leading to students being awarded the pre-registration qualification. Since then, further changes have included the addition of the option to study for a BSc in Operating Department Practice, which includes being able to achieve this qualification via the apprenticeship route (CODP 2009, 2012).

Like all changes, initially there were some concerns that these developments represented an erosion of the deep-seated relationship between learning and the practical aspects of the ODP role, but there has been a subsequent and significant shift in culture and attitude. The advantages and benefits of the courses have become more apparent, the most observable being the increase in opportunities for ODPs to widen their scope of practice, both inside and outside their traditional location, in perioperative environments (CODP 2010). ODPs are no longer confined to the anaesthetic rooms as they once were. Increasingly, they are employed in more diverse roles, both in the healthcare sector and other areas. This has been, in part, due to recognition of ODPs' unique clinical skills, specialist knowledge and adaptability, as well as the skills and attributes associated with 'graduates', such as leadership, problem-solving, decision-making and emotional intelligence. These additional, and valued, associated attributes, including professional responsibilities, such as knowing the importance of CPD, have been integrated into the pre-registration healthcare programmes.

The changes to the pre-registration education of ODPs occurred around the time that the role attained the status of a profession in 2004, to be regulated by the Health and Care Professions Council (HCPC). One of the most significant changes, which came as part of this statutory regulation by the HCPC, was the introduction of mandatory CPD for all registrants from July 2006 onwards. The rationale for its introduction was that it is an important dimension of professionals' self-regulation and is linked to the role's primary function, which is protecting the health and well-being of members of the public (HCPC 2004). For this reason, and in accordance with the HCPC's 'Standards of conduct, performance and ethics', it is the responsibility of registered ODPs to ensure that their knowledge, skills and performance in their areas of practice are of a high quality and up to date (HCPC 2016). The importance of engaging in career-long, self-directed learning as a mechanism for maintaining fitness to practice is also clearly stated in the HCPC's 'Standards of proficiency: Operating Department Practitioners' (HCPC 2023).

Professionalization and CPD

We often hear the phrase, 'Trust me, I'm a professional', but what does it mean to be a professional and, in particular, a healthcare professional? What defines someone as an ODP? What sets ODPs apart from other occupational groups?

In the literature, health and social care professions are often referred to as 'caring professions' (Ellis and Hogard 2021). When reviewing the definitions for what a 'profession' is in the literature, a number of characteristics are distinguishable, ones that apply to ODPs. Each profession has:

- a distinct body of knowledge;
- monitored and validated education and training programmes required to qualify;

- a register of members and self-regulation through the relevant professional body;
- codes of conduct and ethics, and participation in a subculture sustained by professional associations;
- engages in CPD, to demonstrate continued competence and fitness to practise.

A number of these characteristics have been explored in Chapter 3, about professional practice, but note the final defining characteristic of a profession listed here, which is the requirement to engage in CPD. According to Friedman (2013), undertaking CPD is a key component in being a professional, and the means by which we keep our knowledge and skills up to date when set against a dynamically changing environment. Thus, the nature of and relationship with CPD for a profession is extended, as it is an intrinsic part of ODPs' professional identity and everyday working practices. It is also a process that not only enables ODPs to re-register with the HCPC but also is a measure of an ongoing competence and fitness to practice, and to meet the challenges of a changing healthcare system. Further, failure to submit evidence of CPD and learning activities on request, or to demonstrate a sufficient range of CPD, can result in suspension or removal from the register. Therefore, the relevance and importance of CPD, as well as the responsibility owed to colleagues and patients to keep up to date, cannot be over-emphasized.

Why CPD?

New knowledge, new procedures, new processes and new environments bring about new thinking, new actions and new ideas. Therefore, a professional person who does not understand and implement the need for CPD in a lifelong learning world is not only standing still but is also falling behind (Keith and Longworth 2017).

It is recognized that initial training and qualifications alone are insufficient to meet the needs and expectations of a changing society during a person's working life (Roscoe 2002). Indeed, the knowledge and skills with which each ODP begins their career have a short 'shelf life', with estimates that the lifespan of that knowledge, particularly in medicine and healthcare, is approximately two years. Further, as we live in a digital age, the impact of digital healthcare technologies across many healthcare environments, including operating theatres, affect the healthcare workforce as we need to acquire the necessary digital literacy skills to use equipment and systems effectively and safely (HEE 2019).

Many ODPs, especially those who trained at the time of the older (pre-diploma) awards, may not have formalized their CPD or recorded it appropriately, as their CPD activities may have been centred on the requirements of their immediate roles, responsibilities or needs. However, as the role has expanded and responsibilities have increased, this has led to the expectation that ODPs will take responsibility for managing both their career pathways and planning their own learning needs to ensure that their knowledge and skills remain current. Participation in CPD has thus become an integral part of ODPs' practice as it serves to fulfil a number of requirements.

Defining lifelong learning and CPD

Lifelong learning and CPD are both well-established principles that drive the ongoing education, training and development of many healthcare professions (Department of Health (DH) 2004), including ODPs. The two terms are often used interchangeably and do share some common characteristics, both serving to encompass a full range of learning activities contributing to personal development as well as benefiting wider social dimensions. However, it is important to consider the distinction between them so that ODPs meet the requirements of both their profession and their employment.

'Lifelong learning' is a broad term that is used by governments and other organizations to describe learning that meets the challenges of globalization that have presented themselves as part of the emergence of a knowledge-based economy. From the National Health Service's (NHS) perspective, therefore, lifelong learning is considered crucial to enabling the delivery of the government's vision of a world-class healthcare service (DH 2012). The NHS displays its commitment to lifelong learning principles through its many policies and plans that reiterate the valuable contribution learning, in all its forms, makes to practitioners' everyday working practices, particularly when it comes to contributing to the quality of patient care, and ensuring the effective and efficient provision of services (Imison et al. 2016; DHSC 2019).

The importance placed on training, education and development is perhaps more evident following the Francis report (2013), as the NHS has since been placed under increased scrutiny as a result of its findings. Regular audits of hospitals by the Care Quality Commission (CQC) monitor patient service, quality and experiences, including in relation to operating theatres, with education and training forming a major component of the recommendations of these audits. 'The NHS Constitution for England' (DH 2021) highlights the commitment to providing staff with personal development opportunities so that they can undertake their roles and it has been recognized that there is a link between healthcare education and the delivery of safe patient care. The NHS has also emphasized the importance of teaching non-technical skills, such as communication and teamworking, to directly address patient safety issues. This is evident in the perioperative environment through the introduction of the World Health Organization's 'WHO guidelines for safe surgery 2009' (WHO 2009) and human factors training (NHS England 2013), which are both high-profile initiatives with a specific focus on operating department practice.

CPD is a process by which ODPs regularly demonstrate that they are meeting their professional responsibilities and maintaining their competence and fitness to practise. It provides a framework that enables ODPs to meet the growing demand for quality, competence and accountability, and ensures that patients receive the best possible care. In addition, it serves to help ODPs to respond to ongoing changes in their own practice areas as they feature in the wider challenges of healthcare provision.

Stop and think

Think about your current role and reflect on these questions.

What organizational, departmental or procedural changes (if any) have you experienced during the past year?

How have they affected you and how have you adapted to those changes?

Were there any training or support mechanisms in place to help you meet those changes?

Focusing on CPD?

Although CPD shares commonalities with lifelong learning, and occupies a unique position on the lifelong learning continuum, it possesses a number of distinct features. Whereas lifelong learning is portrayed as being inclusive of all learning 'from cradle to grave', CPD is a process of structured, specific learning and development, determined and undertaken by an individual during the 'practitioner's working life' (Megginson and Whittaker 2007: 5) and involves aspects of reflection, action and, importantly, application to practice. Furthermore, it has become synonymous with professionalism and the development of a professional identity, with the learning governed by professional standards.

The term 'continuing professional development' (CPD) is attributed to Richard Gardner, who was responsible for professional development in the building professions at York University during the 1970s. His intention was to introduce a framework of professional development with the intention of re-establishing the links between education and practice, which he saw as lacking in post-qualified practising professionals (Gardner 1978). Gardner also recognized the multidimensional nature of knowledge, which is that it encompasses technical, process-related, professional and tacit knowledge, but the informal, work-based and incidental learning we engage in through our everyday practices is also of importance. CPD, in his view, is also a formal and more public way to organize what professionals do informally as part of their working lives. Recognition of the value of CPD led to the adoption and introduction of CPD policies across a number of professional bodies during the late 1990s.

A wealth of definitions of CPD can be found in the literature, from Bubb and Earley's (2007: 3) elegantly simple and straightforward description of it as a process that 'encompasses all formal and informal learning that enables individuals to improve their practice' to more in-depth and profession-specific ones. The professional regulator for ODPs, the HCPC (2012), defines CPD as:

> a range of learning activities through which professionals maintain and develop throughout their career to ensure that they retain their capacity to practise safely, effectively and legally within their evolving scope of practice.

This profession-generic definition predominantly focuses on the individual practitioner, their responsibilities and obligations to practise in their defined roles according to 'Standards of conduct, performance and ethics' (HCPC 2016).

While in other professions the requirement is to undertake a specific number of hours or gather a designated number of points as evidence of their CPD activities, the HCPC decided to opt for a less prescriptive approach. The view was taken that, due to the differing nature of the individual registrants and their diverse roles, each practitioner will be able to dedicate different amounts of time to learning (HCPC 2004). There is also the possibility that, if it had followed other professions, learning could become a points-gathering exercise, which, in turn, would negate any meaning or value attached to the learning.

Although broadness and flexibility exist regarding the 'range of learning activities' deemed relevant by the HCPC, it further acknowledges the variations in ODPs' individual roles, responsibilities and learning needs, while still adhering to the need to meet professional standards. The HCPC's definition also alludes to the wider contexts of practice opening up and the increase in links with other areas, both inside and outside the organization, as ODPs' roles and scope of practice move beyond the traditional, defined boundaries. Indeed, the phrase 'evolving scope of practice' signposts not only individuals' potential achievements but also acknowledges and sanctions the fact that the healthcare workforce and practices are changing. This highlights that ODPs, as knowledgeable workers, are required to adjust to new and evolving situations as government targets and initiatives challenge their current roles and responsibilities. And as changes are becoming more frequent, the importance of measurable CPD becomes more imperative.

Although we 'know' or have our own ideas as to what constitutes CPD, and recognize it as an accepted and intrinsic component of our professional identity and practice, research concludes that CPD is not a straightforward concept. Its ambiguous nature results from the 'definitional variety between professional associations' with respect to their body of professional knowledge and practice (Friedman 2013) and the dynamically changing traditions of professionalism. This is further compounded by the myriad interchangeable terms – 'continuing (professional) education', 'CPD' and 'lifelong learning', among others – each with a variety of conflicting definitions. The one distinguishing feature that appears to separate the terms hinges on the value attributed to particular learning activities, with formal academic learning being favoured particularly, as it carries more weight and credibility than informal and work-based learning.

Although definitions of CPD vary, they share some common, fundamental features: it should be continual, profession-focused and broad-based (Kennie 1998). The following principles should also have been built into it so that the learning:

- is patient-centred;
- is the responsibility the individual practitioner to manage;
- involves participation on behalf of the relevant stakeholders (the practitioner, organization, education provider, professional regulator);
- is educationally effective;
- meets the learning needs, which are clearly stated and reflect the wider objectives of the organization, locally and nationally;

- enhances the knowledge and skills of the practitioner;
- involves the application of evidence-based research and practice;
- is an integral part of everyday working practice rather than seen as a burden.

The final principle is an important one and reiterates how ODPs should view CPD. It should not be about doing just enough to meet the requirements of registration, nor should it be left to the last minute. It should be, as Kennie states, a continual and ongoing process that becomes embedded in OPDs' everyday practices and, therefore, is something to be embraced because the benefits of engaging in learning prove to be bountiful and productive.

Exploring the benefits of CPD

So what *are* the advantages or benefits of engaging in CPD? Just as there are endless differing views and definitions of CPD, the benefits of engaging in learning are wide-reaching. For ODPs, as well as the individual, the organization, the professional body and, most importantly, the patients and service users are all beneficiaries of the learning and development that take place.

Each ODP will have their own perceptions of what CPD can 'do' for them and their own reasons for undertaking particular learning activities. These may be linked to immediate short-term goals, such as training in how to use new equipment or updating knowledge to incorporate the guidance for current policies into practice. Longer-term professional development goals may include career-orientated needs, such as promotion, extending their role or qualifying for advanced practitioner roles. In your own professional context, engaging in CPD should be of benefit in terms of your own development but, equally, your new skills can be focused on and directed towards caring for your patients. Furthermore, it serves to ensure that all carry out their roles and responsibilities safely and effectively, as defined by their scope of practice.

Stop and think

Think about a recent learning activity you have undertaken.

What was its purpose? What have you learnt from it? In what way has it benefited you?

In what way has your learning benefited your patients?

Sadler-Smith et al. (2000) identify three main reasons for undertaking CPD: mobility, maintenance and survival. Evidence from across the literature indicates other similar motives: personal development, career or job satisfaction, increased confidence in carrying out our various roles and the updating of knowledge and skills (Pool et al. 2016). For some practitioners, CPD is synonymous with 'credentialism' (Morgan et al. 2008), which is when obtaining academic qualifications makes it possible to achieve a 'simple selection for recruitment and promotion'

(Hewison et al. 2000: 270). Conversely, some ODPs may view CPD as a necessary evil, 'to prevent them going backwards . . . rather than to advance themselves' (Murphy et al. 2006: 378) or for 'fear of being overtaken by less experienced but more academically qualified staff' (Dowswell et al. 1997: 546). Rothwell and Arnold (2005) focus on professional dimensions, citing 'avoiding losing one's license to practise' and 'affirming the individual as a good professional' (Rothwell and Arnold 2005: 29), which are equally valid reasons for undertaking learning.

Moving away from learning simply as a means for personal gain, such as promotion and to remain registered, regularly engaging in CPD activities is acknowledged to have a number of further benefits. It can help to build confidence in your role and increase your credibility as a registered ODP, as well as develop coping mechanisms to manage the changing environment and update your skill set. Regularly reviewing your learning and reflection on this will highlight gaps in your knowledge and experience that will enable you to take responsibility for developing a learning structure. Linking learning to your annual appraisal enables you to also measure your achievements as an individual. Learning in your practice area and alongside colleagues promotes better staff morale and develops a motivated workforce and that, ultimately, results in enhanced patient care. As organizations have shifted responsibility for learning on to individual practitioners, the ability of the individual to take on that responsibility and plan their own professional development is seen as a significant strength. Having a learning framework also aids the organization in its planning of the learning needs of the workforce, so that it aligns this with its wider business objectives, which helps to link theory to practice.

Motivation almost certainly plays a part in our pursuit of learning. According to Smith and Spurling (2005: 2), motivation is a multifaceted concept and, loosely defined, is 'the personal experience of keenness for pursuing an intended action or goal'. A number of factors are recognized as being responsible for directing individuals in their pursuit of an intended goal. McGivney (1990) cites three motivating factors that may influence an ODP's pursuit of a particular learning activity: extrinsic, intrinsic and social.

'Extrinsic factors' are external and varied in the healthcare sector but generally are driven by government policies and dictates that determine service needs, local initiatives and target setting. Extrinsic factors that directly influence individuals primarily relate to incentives, rewards or positive reinforcement for engaging in a particular practice or goal. In the context of learning, external factors that provide motivation include meeting organizational requirements as part of your employment status, such as completion of statutory and mandatory training, and maintaining competence to practice in your professional remit.

'Intrinsic factors' derive from an internal desire, so are considered stronger and more enduring than extrinsic factors (Rogers 2002: 95). Intrinsic factors emanate from the individual through a need to succeed or survive (Maslow 1954). These are often related to your professional identity or a sense of belonging to a particular group as a way of establishing yourself among your peers and colleagues. This in itself echoes the strong relationship that learning and CPD have for professionals.

Motivation is further governed by social factors, such as the expectation of rewards or success, which could include job satisfaction, benefiting patient care or promotion.

Stop and think

What motivates you in your choice of learning activities?

Planning and managing CPD

How do we plan and manage our CPD? According to Megginson and Whittaker (2007), successful learning is founded on a mutual relationship between employer and employee in which both parties benefit from the learning undertaken. In this situation, an ODP who is proactive in determining their own learning needs will be empowered by the process and so learning becomes 'an integral part of all work activity' (Megginson and Whittaker 2007: 5).

The majority of our learning activities are determined by internal processes, although some learning can be ad hoc. However, the appraisal system or personal development plan is often the best way to give some thought to your learning needs for the coming year. This should involve a discussion with your line manager (or someone who is in a suitable position to advise and direct your goals), who may make suggestions regarding your development and these may reflect wider organizational strategies. This process can be beneficial for members of staff at all grades for reviewing their current role, responsibilities practice and performance, including a consideration of future requirements. It can be a useful tool for looking at yourself as a whole and can serve to highlight any areas for future personal development. It can also help you focus on the next year – what is going to change, such as the introduction of new services, which may require further training for all staff. Use it as a tool to help you.

You may already have a clear plan for the learning activities you wish to access. You may be considering promotion and want to know what is required of you to be eligible to apply. You may want support in extending your scope of practice by applying for advanced roles or taking on a specialist lead role in your specific area of practice. If you are thinking of applying for study leave or funding, it may be beneficial to consult your local education and training policy as each organization will have different processes. It may also provide insight into the organization's education strategy. There is a tendency for learning activities to be prioritized that relate to wider organizational objectives. Your local training and education policy should clearly indicate which learning activities are considered to be a priority and so may be better supported in financial terms or time allowed for study.

Although the appraisal process may appear time-consuming and perhaps requests are not fulfilled, it can be a valuable exercise as it contributes to developing the organization's training needs analysis. This, in turn, feeds into the actions of wider stakeholders and commissioning processes for learning activities locally, in-house or in partnership with local HEI and the commissioners of education.

Which forms of learning constitute CPD?

A common myth is that CPD is all about formal, academic study. This is not the case. Learning under the CPD umbrella, and advocated by the HCPC in its definition that we looked at earlier in this chapter, takes an inclusive approach that serves to incorporate formal, informal, work-based and incidental learning. In its guide to CPD, the HCPC (2004) provides a comprehensive, but not prescriptive, list of learning activities and offers guidance and ideas under five headings: work-based learning, professional activity, formal/educational, self-directed learning and other. From a practitioner's perspective, and in accordance with the HCPC's requirements for CPD, it is also considered good practice to have a broad spread of learning activities.

In adopting a 'context-driven' and outcomes-based approach to CPD, the HCPC acknowledges that ODPs' ability to engage in learning activities is determined by a number of issues. ODPs' roles, responsibilities and practice interests vary; learning opportunities will differ from one organization to another, as will the learning styles and preferences of individual practitioners. Furthermore, it is important to remember that ODPs' learning needs will also vary depending on how long they have been qualified and the position they hold in their department – the learning needs of a newly qualified ODP will differ considerably from those of a senior practitioner with management responsibilities, for example. In addition, your practice context, scope of practice and the organization's wider service needs will also influence how you engage in particular learning activities. An ODP practising in the anaesthetic remit will have different learning needs from an ODP who practises primarily as a surgical practitioner, and both will differ further from those ODPs who practise outside the normal theatre environment.

Stop and think

You may be considering promotion or know of forthcoming opportunities for development.

Are you in a position to apply for those opportunities?

What do you need to be doing to enable you to apply and be successful?

Formal learning

Merriam et al. (2007: 29) define formal learning as 'highly institutionalized, bureaucratic, curriculum driven and formally recognized with grades, diplomas and certificates'. This epitomizes the generally held view of both learning and education that takes place in specific buildings or institutions, at specific times during a learner's lifetime and between distinctive parties – teachers educating and students being educated (Curtis and Pettigrew 2010: 154).

As noted earlier, CPD is not all about formal or academic learning, although gaining a degree is held in high regard, particularly in the healthcare sector, as it is considered to enable practitioners to be more effective in delivering patient care (Davey and Robinson 2002). For some ODPs, embarking on post-registration study (such as a top-up degree, a master's or doctoral pathway) may be a personal goal. For others, it may be a requirement of their current role or an important aspect of their future career development. A number of different apprenticeship programmes are also available for qualified practitioners, so that may be an option to explore.

For those ODPs who may not be motivated or disposed towards completing a full academic award, there are other options available. As part of your personal and professional development, you may be required to undertake training to become a practice educator or supervisor, which will enable you to teach and assess student ODPs during their clinical placements. Involvement in supporting students also constitutes professional activity in the HCPC's list of CPD activities. You may then consider developing your skills in the education field and enrol on a specific teacher training module. Embarking on this module may also provide the incentive to continue studying at this level.

You might also find that your own organization runs recognized in-house formal courses, such as immediate and advanced life support. Some provide management and leadership programmes, the aim of which is to support newly promoted staff or those wishing to progress in their careers. Your personal interests may lead you to take on additional link or lead roles, such as robotic surgery, simulation, infection control, health and safety or be a manual handling trainer. Alternatively, have you considered becoming a cascade trainer for medical equipment? These lead roles will often be supported and run by your organization but can be supplemented by formal programmes delivered by external providers.

Work-based learning activities

Not everyone is disposed towards formal learning, preferring practical, hands-on and work-based activities that are directly applicable to their clinical roles. In the literature, workplace learning usually comes under the 'informal learning' umbrella, due to its unstructured nature. As a result, it often receives less attention and is perceived as having less credibility than learning associated with formal qualifications. But work-based learning is an extremely valuable, easily accessible and beneficial form of learning that is not to be underestimated.

Stephen Billett (2020) is a champion of work-based learning and campaigns for it to be established as a recognized form of education in its own right. The workplace and day-to-day practices can create a wealth of learning opportunities. Although no formal curriculum exists for this learning strategy, the repetitive and ritualistic nature of work practices develops its own evolving and continual curriculum. Every day can present new and exciting challenges and opportunities for learning – new equipment, new techniques and new procedures provide a richness of new knowledge and skills. Operating theatres are acknowledged to be truly interprofessional and multidisciplinary environments, where our current and expanding roles can often bring us into contact with other healthcare practitioners who provide opportunities for learning, sharing new ideas and best practices. As a consequence, our immediate workplace assumes a more prominent position as a learning environment. As Eraut (2006: 10) points out in his exploration of professional knowledge and competence, 'professionals continually learn on the job because their work entails engagement in a succession of cases, problems or projects which they have to learn about'.

It is likely that you will supervise other staff and students coming into your department. As well as teaching and supporting them, you might also learn from them. The wealth of knowledge held in a workplace, particularly by the experienced practitioners, provides opportunities for discussion, clinical supervision, shadowing, mentoring, networking and cascade learning that are all recognized as valued CPD activities (HCPC 2017). The merits of work-based learning rest in its direct applicability to everyday practice, which means that highly specific, as well as transferable, knowledge and skills are developed and applied directly to patient care.

Another term you may come across is 'self-directed learning'. This can take different forms and is a valuable way to learn. For example, how many journals do you see lying around in the staff room or left elsewhere? Have you ever picked them up and read some of the articles? What did you think of them? Have you discussed changes in practice with colleagues? Have you been prompted to look up a new or unfamiliar procedure on the Internet? Has one of your students asked you a question that you cannot answer?

Reflective practice is another valuable learning activity, and one that is discussed in depth in Chapter 5, on reflection.

When learning becomes part of our everyday practice, it contributes to our motivation, interest and the sustainability of learning as we frequently engage in such learning practices. Rather than waiting for learning opportunities to come to you, you may become motivated to actively seek out or set up learning activities in your own department, such as journal clubs, case study presentations, departmental meetings and clinical audits. Have you considered writing an article for a professional journal? Have you reported back on any training you have recently undertaken or been involved in?

Planning and managing your CPD

It is recognized that the transition from student ODP to newly qualified practitioner can be daunting and challenging. Support and guidance during the first six months to a year can be of great benefit, and many hospital trusts have adopted a preceptorship framework for this purpose (NHS England 2022). The aims of this programme of support and study, which is structured for all newly qualified (non-medical) healthcare professionals, are to enhance the competence and confidence of registered practitioners to help them to:

> translate and embed their knowledge into everyday practice, grow in confidence and have the best possible start to their careers (NHS England 2022).

A possible pathway for a newly qualified ODP during their first year could include:

- a trust, local induction or preceptorship programme;
- statutory and mandatory training;

- speciality specific learning, completion of specific competences;
- rotation of anaesthesia, surgery and post-anaesthetic care;
- medical devices training;
- blood transfusion training – including cell salvage;
- immediate or advanced life support training;
- supporting healthcare students in their practice, which may include formal mentorship training, or practice educator and supervisor training;
- appraisal and planning learning for the next year.

This list is not meant to be prescriptive, but it does offer some possible suggestions for development during the first year as a newly qualified ODP, leading into the two-year audit period for registration. Just because someone is newly qualified does not mean that they are not already thinking ahead. It is important to remember, however, that what will be ideal CPD, particularly during the first year (and, indeed, during your later career), will depend on the ODP's role and areas of practice, as well as the requirements of their department and organization.

So what about someone who has been qualified a few years? As your career progresses your requirements for CPD will reflect your developing role, responsibilities, experiences and interests. How can you continue to meet your professional responsibilities? Here are some suggestions:

- complete statutory and mandatory training;
- reflect in and on your practice;
- ensure you go on rotation to various specialisms to update or enhance your skills;
- shadow a member of staff or go on a secondment;
- deputize for senior staff or colleagues;
- undergo clinical supervision;
- be a link person for infection control, health and safety or diabetes;
- develop a specialist interest area or become a lead practitioner;
- be a cascade trainer for medical equipment;
- mentor and teach students;
- be a preceptor for newly qualified staff;
- undertake to be a surgical first assistant (extended scope of practice), surgical care practitioner education, advanced care practitioner or anaesthesia associate;
- undertake appraisals for 'junior' staff;
- undertake a clinical audit and research;
- undertake further formal academic awards;
- implement or change aspects of your practice;
- get leadership or management experience or responsibilities;
- consider emergency scenarios, simulation, skills and drills;
- complete online CPD training programmes or resources;
- read and review journal articles.

CPD and the re-registration process

As you will be aware, to continue to practise and use the protected title of ODP, you are required to renew your registration every two years. This process helps the HCPC to demonstrate that their registrants are maintaining their competence, knowledge and skills and meeting its standards.

The HCPC randomly selects a percentage of the ODP registrants to submit their CPD profile, detailing the learning activities that they have undertaken during the previous two years. The HCPC states that only those registrants who have been on the register for a full two years will be eligible for selection for an audit (HCPC 2017). This allows individuals sufficient time to undertake CPD and meet the HCPC's specific requirements.

The HCPC's 'Your guide to our standards of continuing professional development' (2012) requires you to:

- maintain an accurate and up-to-date record of your CPD activities;
- demonstrate that your CPD activities are a mixture of learning relevant to your current and future practice;
- ensure that your CPD contributes to the quality of your practice and delivery of services to patients;
- ensure that the CPD activities benefit patients and service users;
- on request, present your written profile, complete with supporting evidence explaining how you meet the standards.

What to do if you are selected to submit your CPD profile

So, what if I am selected for audit by the HCPC? First of all, *do not panic*! The HCPC's website has all the support information you need to help you complete your CPD profile, including videos, webinars, sample profiles and reflective templates.

Stop and think

If you were selected to submit your CPD profile today, how confident are you that you would meet the standards?

Make a list of the learning activities you have done in the past three months.

Do you have any evidence to support your learning?

Second, you need to have kept a good record of the learning activities you have undertaken in the time period specified by the HCPC. It is important to remember that keeping a learning log, writing things down and recording your thoughts about your learning and experiences are all an essential part of undertaking CPD.

We all have different ways we prefer to keep such records. Some keep a diary of the particular operating lists we do, procedures we have scrubbed in for, any incidental or work-based learning activities we have engaged in. Another option is to keep a portfolio of your training and development, complete with any certificates of in-house learning you may have completed. Your line manager or education lead should also have a record of your ongoing training in your department, particularly statutory and mandatory training, which is usually kept for audit purposes. Remember, certificates of attendance are valuable evidence, but more importantly, what have you learnt from the study, teaching session? How does it relate to your practice?

Third, however you choose to keep your record of learning activities, it is imperative that it is up to date and can be submitted as evidence if you are selected to do so. Consider it good practice to update your CPD records on a regular basis – weekly or monthly – not leave it to the last minute, so you find yourself scrambling around for certificates or evidence of learning that you have undertaken.

Colleagues who have been selected by the HCPC to submit their profile who did not do this reported that the most challenging part was finding the dates they undertook training and the required supporting evidence. Personally, I use a mixture of methods for recording my learning: I have a diary for recording any day-to-day activities, a portfolio of training certificates and, more recently, I have been entering my learning activities into the electronic CPD profile template that can be downloaded from the HCPC's website. So, if I am selected by the HCPC for audit I am at least part-way there, and meeting Standards One and Five for CPD.

To satisfy the requirements for submitting your profile, you need to provide the following.

- A summary of your current practice area (in a maximum of 500 words). This should include a description of your role and the type of work you undertake, whether you practise primarily in anaesthetics, surgery or recovery, or you regularly move between the three areas of perioperative practice. Your job description may help you with these aspects. You may move between particular specialties or be highly specialized in one area. Who do you communicate with on a daily basis? Do you work in a day-case surgical unit or a large acute Trust with trauma centre status? Perhaps you practise in a non-traditional area, such as sterile services, pre-admissions, critical care, research and audit, quality, safety and improvement or on the transplant team?
- A personal statement (a maximum of 1,500 words). Select a number of CPD activities (between three and five) that you undertook during the specified time period. To fulfil the requirements for profile submission and meet Standard Two, these must be a mixture of learning activities, ones that reflect your current practice and future intentions. Once you have selected your CPD activities that best reflect your own personal learning, ask yourself the questions in the 'Stop and think box'. These will help you to achieve Standards Three and Four.

Stop and think

How has your learning benefited and improved the quality of your practice?

How has your learning benefited your patients and wider service users?

How does your learning enable you to practise safely and effectively?

How does your CPD relate to your changing work practices?

Barriers to learning

The financial and other difficulties experienced in the NHS have served to create a less-than-ideal environment to engage in CPD. Research indicates that there are several barriers to CPD, including a lack of time coupled with an increased workload, lack of understanding of issues relating to CPD, a shortage of staff and lack of management support (Summers 2015; Walter and Terry 2021).

We have all probably experienced these issues at some point and it can be extremely frustrating, especially when other healthcare professionals receive 'protected learning time', such as doctors and dentists. So how can you keep up to date with our CPD responsibilities and ensure that your knowledge, skills and performance are of a high quality, while overcoming such barriers to learning? Here are some suggestions and examples of possible CPD activities.

- Be prepared to do some CPD in your own time. You may be able to claim the time in lieu.
- Use your time effectively. Do you have theatre downtime or audit meetings? Do you regularly attend department meetings or undertake a form of clinical supervision?
- If you have the opportunity, have you considered setting up and running training or study days yourself?
- Be flexible. If you are funded for a course, you may be required to study in your own time. Conversely, you may be offered study time if you fund or part-fund your study. This will depend on your organization's policy.
- Online or e-learning modules are widely available. Some HEIs deliver the practice educator training online, for example, and the Blood Transfusion Service has good e-learning packages, particularly on cell salvage.
- Medical companies and representatives are often willing to give up their time to deliver specific training sessions. Some have teaching and learning packages.
- What is available in your department? Some medical staff may be willing to do some teaching or training sessions as part of their own development.

Conclusion

The aim of this chapter has been to explore the concepts and practices relating to CPD in the specific context of operating department practice. Mandatory CPD is a relatively new concept, but one that has become an integral aspect of ODPs' professional identity and professional practice. There is flexibility, however, and personal choice in how you learn and the types of learning you decide to engage in. Remember that the learning you undertake should be relevant to your current or future role and be of benefit to your practice, patients and service users.

Key points

- CPD is an essential component of operating department practice and should be integral to the role of every ODP.
- CPD serves to benefit the learner, the organization and, most importantly, the patients.
- CPD can be achieved using various methods and ODPs should undertake a variety of different of activities.
- ODPs must be able to submit evidence of their CPD if selected for audit by the HCPC, in the advised format.

References and further reading

Billett, S. (2020) *Learning in the Workplace: Strategies for Effective Practice*. Abingdon: Routledge.

Bubb, S. and Earley, P. (2007) *Leading and Managing Continuing Professional Development*, 2nd edn. London: Paul Chapman.

College of Operating Department Practitioners (CODP) (2009) Standards, recommendations and guidance for mentors and practice placements: Supporting pre-registration education in operating department practice provision. London: CODP.

College of Operating Department Practitioners (CODP) (2010) Framing the future role and function of Operating Department Practitioners: Discussion paper. London: CODP.

College of Operating Department Practitioners (CODP) (2012) Notice of withdrawal of the pre-registration DipHE Operating Department Practice Curriculum, *Technic*, 3(6): 7.

Curtis, W. and Pettigrew, A. (2010) *Education Studies: Reflective Reader*. Exeter: Learning Matters.

Davey, B. and Robinson, S. (2002) Taking a degree after qualifying as a registered general nurse: Constraints and effects, *Nurse Education Today*, 22: 624–32.

Department of Health (DH) (2004) Learning for delivery: Making connections between post qualification learning/continuing professional development and service planning. London: DH.

Department of Health (DH) (2012) Liberating the NHS: Developing the healthcare workforce: from design to delivery. London: DH. Available at: https://assets.publishing.service.gov.uk/government/uploads/system/uploads/attachment_data/file/216421/dh_132087.pdf (accessed November 2022).

Department of Health (DH) (2021) The NHS Constitution for England. London: DH. Available at: www.gov.uk/government/publications/the-nhs-constitution-for-england/the-nhs-constitution-for-england (accessed November 2022).

Department of Health and Social Care (DHSC) (2019) Department of Health and Social Care mandate to Health Education England: April 2018 to March 2019. London: DHSC. Available at: https://assets.publishing.service.gov.uk/government/uploads/system/uploads/attachment_data/file/781757/DHSC_mandate_to_Health_Education_England_-_April_2018_to_March_2019.pdf (accessed November 2022).

Dowswell, T., Hewison, J. and Millare, B. (1997) Joining the learning society and working in the NHS: Some issues, *Journal of Education Policy*, 12(6): 539–50.

Ellis, R. and Hogard, E. (2021) *Professional Identity in the Caring Professions*. Abingdon: Routledge.

Eraut, M. (2006) *Developing Professional Knowledge and Competence*. London: Falmer.

Francis, R. (2013) Report of the Mid Staffordshire NHS Foundation Trust public inquiry: Executive summary. HC 947. London: The Stationery Office. Available at: https://assets.publishing.service.gov.uk/government/uploads/system/uploads/attachment_data/file/279124/0947.pdf (accessed November 2022).

Freidman, A. (2013) *Continuing Professional Development: Lifelong Learning of Millions*. New York: Routledge.

Gardner, R. (1978) Policy on continuing education: A report with recommendations for action. York: University of York.

Health and Care Professions Council (HCPC) (2004) Continuing professional development: Consultation paper. London: HCPC.

Health and Care Professions Council (HCPC) (2012) Your guide to our standards of continuing professional development. London: HCPC.

Health and Care Professions Council (HCPC) (2016) Standards of conduct, performance and ethics. London: HCPC.

Health and Care Professions Council (HCPC) (2017) Continuing professional development and your registration. London: HCPC.

Health and Care Professions Council (HCPC) (2023) Standards of proficiency: Operating Department Practitioners. London: HCPC.

Health Education England (HEE) (2019) The Topol review: Preparing the healthcare workforce to deliver the digital future. London: HEE.

Hewison, J., Dowswell, T. and Millar, B. (2000) Changing patterns of training provision in the National Health Service: An overview, in F. Coffield (ed.), *Differing Visions of a Learning Society: Research Findings Volume 1*. Bristol: Policy Press.

Imison, C., Castle-Clarke, S. and Watson, R. (2016) Reshaping the workforce to deliver the care patients need: Research report. London: Nuffield Trust.

Keith, D.W. and Longworth, N. (2017) *Lifelong Learning*. Abingdon: Routledge.

Kennie, T.J.M. (1998) The growing importance of CPD. *Continuing Professional Development*, 1: 160–9.

Maslow, A. (1954) *Motivation and Personality*. New York: Harper.

McGivney, V. (1990) *Education's for Other People: Access to Education for Non-Participant Adults*. Leicester: National Institute of Adult Continuing Education.

Megginson, D. and Whittaker, V. (2007) *Continuing Professional Development*. London: Chartered Institute of Personnel and Development.

Merriam, S., Caffarella, R. and Baumgartner, L. (2007) *Learning in Adulthood: A Comprehensive Guide*, 3rd edn. New York: John Wiley & Sons, Inc.

Morgan, A., Cullinane, J. and Pye. M. (2008) Continuing professional development: Rhetoric and practice in the NHS, *Journal of Education and Work*, 21(3): 233–48.

Murphy, C., Cross, C. and McGuire, D. (2006) The motivation of nurses to participate in continuing professional education, *Journal of European Industrial Training*, 30(5): 365–84.

NHS England (2013) Human factors in healthcare: A concordat from the National Quality Board. London: NHS England. Available at: www.england.nhs.uk/wp-content/uploads/2013/11/nqb-hum-fact-concord.pdf (accessed November 2022).

NHS England (2022) National preceptorship framework for nursing. London: NHS England. Available at: www.england.nhs.uk/publication/national-preceptorship-framework-for-nursing (accessed November 2022).

Pool, I.A., Poell, R.F., Berings, M.G.M.C. and ten Cate, O. (2016) Motives and activities for continuing professional development: An exploration of their relationships by integrating literature and interview data, *Nurse Education Today*, 38: 22–8.

Rogers, A. (2002) *Teaching Adults*, 3rd edn. London: Open University Press.

Roscoe, J. (2002) Continuing professional development in higher education, *Human Resource Development International*, 5(1): 3–9.

Rothwell, A. and Arnold, J. (2005) How HR professionals rate 'continuing professional development', *Human Resource Management Journal*, 15(3): 18–32.

Sadler-Smith, E., Allinson, C.W. and Hayes, J. (2000) Learning preferences and cognitive style: Some implications for continuing professional development, *Management Learning*, 31(2): 239–56.

Smith, J. and Spurling A. (2005) *Understanding Motivation for Lifelong Learning.* London: Campaign for Learning.

Summers, A. (2015) Continuing professional development in Australia: Barriers and support, *Journal of Continuing Education in Nursing*, 46(8): 337–9.

Walter, J.K. and Terry, L.M. (2021) Factors influencing nurses' engagement with CPD activities: A systematic review, *British Journal of Nursing*, 30(1): 60–8.

World Health Organization (WHO) (2009) WHO guidelines for safe surgery 2009: Safe surgery saves lives. Geneva: WHO. Available at: www.who.int/teams/integrated-health-services/patient-safety/research/safe-surgery (accessed November 2022).

Index

values
  ethics 186–7
  personal 186
  professional 60, 186–7
VARK modalities 3
veracity 187
vicarious learning 141
vicarious liability 158
virtue ethics 181
vulnerable adult 127, 128–9

ward of court 190
Watson, John B. 139

well-being of teams 89–90
whistle-blowing 168–9
within paradigm research 39
work-based learning 231–2
World Health Organization (WHO)
  definition of health 136
  safe surgery guidelines 117–18,
    224
Wye Valley NHS Trust v. B [2015] 162

X (formerly Twitter) 14

young patients *see* children

Milton Keynes UK
Ingram Content Group UK Ltd.
UKHW020422180324
439575UK00009BA/536